Chapter One - The Reveal

April 18, 2004

People close to me and close to the team had started noticing things and had been asking me questions for a while.

- "Is there something wrong with you?"

- "Do you have a bad back?"

- "Why do you seem so stiff when you walk?"

Those kinds of questions were not going to stop, and even though I dreaded it, I knew that I had to tell them. The day after we lost Game 6 to Detroit 2-0 was the day.

I was so proud to be the associate coach of that Nashville Predators team. This was the pre-lockout and pre-salary cap National Hockey League. The Red Wings had the highest payroll in the league that season at close to $78 million and we were 30th in a 30-team league at just over $23 million. Their team had at least seven players who will eventually make it to the Hall of Fame. It is not easy to play or coach against a team that features players that have the names Lidstrom, Yzerman, Shanahan, Datsyuk, and Zetterberg on the backs of their jerseys. Some of those guys may have been in the latter half of their careers at that point, but they were still an impressive group.

Despite the difference in payrolls, our team fought hard to make the playoffs for the first time in franchise history and we also fought Detroit hard in that series before eventually falling to them in six games.

In the last minute of Game 6, our incredible fans in Nashville were standing and applauding the whole time saluting the effort the team gave all season and specifically in the Detroit series. But instead of celebrating the team's accomplishments, I knew that the time had come for me to reveal what I had been sitting on for the better part of a year.

From the time my coaching career started, my goal was to become a head coach at the NHL level. What I was about to say to the team would spread quickly and I knew that the chances of achieving that dream of becoming a head coach would become very slim.

We were going to have the season-ending team meeting the next day and then everybody would have an individual meeting with head coach Barry Trotz and general manager David Poile. I knew that I had to tell them, so the first thing I did was get up early and I went to the arena.

I said to David, "Can I come see you?"

He didn't know what was going on, and I went upstairs to his office and sat down with him before we had the team meeting. This was a couple of hours before the team was coming in, and I said, "David, there is something I have to tell you… I was diagnosed with Parkinson's a year ago."

He looked at me and said, "Oh my gosh," or something like that. His dad, Bud Poile, had Parkinson's and had died of complications of the disease. We didn't say much because we really didn't know what to say to each other.

I had been diagnosed about 10 months before. My wife Tami and I didn't tell anybody because I was trying to get through the season. We didn't even tell the kids until a few weeks before we told the team.

Following that short meeting with David, I went down and shut the door with Trotzy. I said, "Barry, I was diagnosed with Parkinson's."

All he could say was, "I would never have known. I would have never had any idea."

He is the one closest to me. We see each other every day. He said, "Your brain is still fine, so just do your job and we will get through it."

Then Trotzy said, "You are just going to have to do your work, and I am going to be hard on you. We are just going to get through it and there are no excuses." We just made a pact that we were going to work it out and see how it went.

We then went in and told assistant coach Peter Horachek. It was Peter's first year with the team.

Then I said to Barry and Peter, "Guys I may need some help telling the team because nobody knows and I am a little emotional talking about it right now."

After we had the meeting, I was in pretty good shape, so Trotzy grabbed my arm on one side and I think Peter stood close to me on the other side to make sure I could get through it. I knew that Barry and Peter were great friends, but to have them right there next to me while I was doing one of the most difficult things I had ever done meant more to me than I could ever adequately put into words.

I don't even remember exactly what I said to the team, but I was trying to make a joke, and I said something like, "Guys the reason why I made so many bad passes in practice this year was because I was diagnosed with Parkinson's a year ago and I don't know what is going to happen to me going forward."

Rem Murray was one of the players on that team, and he is truly one of the nicest guys you will ever meet. He had to stop playing about midway through that season because he was diagnosed with a neurological disorder called Dystonia. It caused his head to turn almost all the way to his left shoulder.

I would talk to him and say, 'hang in there' because I knew what he was going through. Not knowing about my diagnosis and trying to look on the bright side, one time he said, "At least I don't have Parkinson's."

He came back after the meeting that day and he felt so badly. He is such a nice guy. He apologized right afterwards. I told him, "You didn't know, It's OK."

That was it, and the guys all came up afterwards to say that they were sorry then everybody dispersed.

After that, the NHL was in the lockout and we didn't see anybody for a year.

Chapter Two - The Discovery

Parkinson's disease is a disorder in the brain. It occurs when certain nerve cells called neurons in a part of the brain called the substantia nigra die or become impaired. Normally, these cells produce a vital chemical known as dopamine. Dopamine allows smooth, coordinated function of the body's muscles and movement. When approximately 80% of the dopamine-producing cells are damaged, the symptoms of Parkinson's disease appear.

Although I have no data to back this up, I believe that I am one of the few Parkinson's patients who was diagnosed by their spouse. Yes, Tami diagnosed my Parkinson's, and no, she is not a neurologist.

One day during the 2002 offseason, she was sitting on the couch in our living room. I was just standing in the doorway, and she could just tell that something was wrong with me. Just by looking at me, she said that I was "from one day to the next" different. It was like I was fine one minute and the next I was completely changed.

Tami had worked in a hospital and she had been around Parkinson's patients, so she was speaking with some experience with the disease. She went on to say that the Spirit had told her that I had Parkinson's.

During my throat surgery earlier that year, Tami had noticed a slight tremor in my right leg while I was lying on the gurney in the hospital.

Tami had fought and plead with me for a year to go to a doctor. I didn't go. I really didn't think that there was anything wrong with me. She could not believe that I would go on denying something like that.

A year later, Tami and I went for a walk around our neighborhood. During the walk, my right arm was not moving; it was just kind of stuck in place.

"Is there something wrong with your arm?" Tami asked.

I told her no, and that it was probably just a pinched nerve from a shoulder surgery that I had years before.

To say that I had dealt with my share of injuries during my playing career would be somewhat of an understatement. In addition to the shoulder surgery, I had five concussions, four broken noses, surgery on both knees, throat surgery, back surgery, two broken legs, and lots of stitches.

When I was still playing, Tami had told me that with all of those injuries that I was going to be a mess and fall apart when I turned 40. She wasn't that far off since I was diagnosed with Parkinson's when I was 44.

Despite my thinking that there was nothing wrong with me, I finally decided to go and get myself checked out by a doctor after the hockey season was over.

The neurologist who diagnosed me did all the walking, touch, and balance tests. He came back into the room and said, "Your right eye isn't blinking Mr. Peterson, you have Parkinson's. Here's the medication." Then he just handed me some Requip, which is one of the medications used to treat Parkinson's.

Tami was, and still is, not a fan of that particular doctor's bedside manner. She says that if she saw him again she would slap him. And she is not kidding. If you think hockey players are tough, hockey wives are even tougher because they have to be. As a player and a coach, you are on the road for half the season, and Murphy's Law seems to always dictate that things go wrong whenever we are out of town. When one of the kids got sick, or the water heater broke, or any other minor emergency occurred, it always happened while I was out of town. Tami took care of whatever needed taking care of when these things happened.

As a player, you always wanted teammates who would have your back out on the ice, so having an enforcer of a wife standing by my side through this entire battle meant so much to me. I am not sure if I would be able to go at this alone, and knowing that Tami would throw down with a neurologist on my behalf makes this fight against Parkinson's feel like a genuine team effort.

After I got the diagnosis, I met Tami in the mall and told her that I had Parkinson's. She responded by saying, "I know you do." She is right about a lot of things, but I really wished that this was one of the few things that she was wrong about.

When I was diagnosed, I did not believe it. I went through a range of emotions, and none of them were good. I was in a very bad place mentally and did not know how to deal with things. There is really no way to prepare yourself for that kind of news.

I really felt I was a bad person, I was a bad husband, I was a bad father, I was all 'woe is me.' I was feeling sorry for myself. I was bitter and angry because I had Parkinson's.

It wasn't fair to me, and it certainly wasn't fair to my family. There is no doubt that hockey is a tough sport and there are definitely risks associated with playing the game, but I made it through my playing career without suffering a catastrophic injury, and now this. I was 44-years-old. Being a coach in my early 40s, about the only thing I should have been concerned about injury or illness-wise would be catching a stray puck that would only require a few stitches to fix.

Parkinson's is about the furthest thing from a stray puck. It is a scary disease, one that has no cure.

With all of the concussions I sustained during my career, it is a logical conclusion that they were the cause of the Parkinson's, but there is really no way of knowing for sure.

One of the concussions was so bad that I had to stay overnight in the hospital. I got out of the hospital the next day, went right to the rink, and got on the bike. I played the next night. We didn't know any better. Thankfully for today's athletes, head injuries are taken much more seriously.

Tami and I decided early on not to tell anyone, since we were afraid that if I used my health insurance, people would know. We didn't know how the insurance worked. We figured they would see all this Parkinson's medication show up and know that I had it.

The medications given to Parkinson's patients attempt to replace the dopamine that their brain does not produce because of the disease. Dopamine controls the body's movement.

By not using my health insurance to pay for the medication, I was taking on a huge financial burden due to the high cost of all of the drugs that are used to try and control the disease.

Tami's parents, Marla and Ralph Stratford, were two of the few people that we told about my diagnosis, and they were extremely generous to help us out by giving us the money to pay for the medication for a year.

Tami didn't know much about Parkinson's, so without telling me, she went to a seminar where a Dr. Hassan spoke. She was crying in the back and he saw her. He spoke to her after and asked her what was wrong. Tami told him the whole story about me being in hockey and we didn't want to tell anybody. We used the money that we received from Tami's parents to pay for the medication that Dr. Hassan prescribed for me. He took care of us for the year we did not tell anyone about my diagnosis.

Chapter Three - A Silent Year

Going almost an entire year without telling anyone that I had Parkinson's really took a toll on me mentally. Once I knew about the diagnosis, I was in shock. It was tough because I didn't have a lot of symptoms. I was still in really good shape, but we were paranoid the whole year. We were afraid someone would see the medication bottles and find out our secret.

Even though I was in good shape, I still became fixated on the little things that I could notice were changing. I couldn't shampoo my hair with my right hand. I couldn't scratch my head with that hand either. I had a hard time tucking in my shirt. In the grand scheme of things, these weren't all that bad, but I just started realizing them more and more. I was consumed with the changes.

While I was focusing on the physical changes that were occurring, I had a hard time focusing on doing my job. I could still do everything that I needed to, but without my head in the right place, I wasn't doing it as well as I should have. I was there, but it was almost like I was just going through the motions. I knew that was the case, but I just couldn't get my head in the right place to change things. And by knowing it, I figured that other people were noticing, which in turn made me more paranoid.

As the hockey season was coming toward its end, I received a phone call that changed me, and it changed me forever.

Cam Neely and I became good friends when we played together in Vancouver. Cam and Michael J. Fox are best friends, so in my time of need, I reached out to Cam through a third party in hopes of speaking with Michael. Even though Cam and I were friends, I was not ready to tell him about the fact that I had Parkinson's at that time. Max Offenberger, who was the team psychologist, was that third party for me. Tami and I reached out to Max to help us try to handle my diagnosis.

Eventually, we wanted his help to find out how she and the kids could deal with it.

Cam lived with Max when he first moved from Vancouver to Boston.

Maxy called Cam and said, "I have somebody that you know that has Parkinson's, but I can't tell you who it is. Can we talk to Michael?"

Cam then called Michael and said that he had a friend that was just diagnosed with Parkinson's, and asked if he could give that friend a call. Cam didn't know it was me, but Maxy's word was good enough for him to try and make the connection.

Michael and I had a tough time getting a hold of each other. One day he called me and for whatever reason where I was driving was a dead cell zone and I started losing him. So I pulled over and drove up this hill. I sat on the top of the hill in this apartment complex and we talked for two hours.

Michael told me about his having to quit playing hockey. He told me about his TV show *Spin City* and about how he would go up and down with his medication. That made doing his job as an actor very difficult. Michael told me about how he kept it from everybody, and then he said to me, "Do me a favor, don't stop doing the things you love doing. Don't stop playing hockey. Don't stop coaching. Don't stop golfing. Even if you look bad at it, don't stop. It's not worth it."

He was great and that was when I turned my attitude around. Michael was great because he told me how things really were. He had experienced the same things that I was going through, so he did not want me to make some of the mistakes he did when he first was diagnosed.

Michael said he made the mistake of hiding the disease and that I shouldn't do that. He told me that we shake, and we tremor, and we walk funny, but we have to get the word out and we have to find a cure. Michael told me, "I am going to find a cure." He went on a rampage about the stem cells and wanting to get taxpayer money for more stem cells as a potential treatment for Parkinson's.

As the conversation came to a close, he told me something that will stick with me for the rest of my life. He said, "Quit feeling sorry for yourself and go do something about it."

Michael told me to just get on with it. At that point, I knew that I had to start telling people the truth.

I knew that I was jeopardizing a lot of things that I had dreamed of doing like becoming a head coach in the NHL, but there was nothing that I could do about it. I had Parkinson's which is non-curable and a progressive disease, so it wasn't going to go away. It was a part of who I was and would be for the rest of my life.

Tami and I started by telling the kids in March.

We had all the kids come into town and we finally told them. When we told them, they were mad at us. They did not talk to us that night because we didn't tell them earlier. Ryan was mad. Kristin was in shock, and Brad asked, "When are you going to die Dad?"

That was hard. It certainly was not a question I was prepared for that day.

Tami and I then made the decision that we were going to tell the team at the end of the season. We knew that after we told the team, the news would spread everywhere.

We made the playoffs that year, so I had to wait a little while following the end of the regular season. Once we lost to Detroit in the playoffs, it was time to stick to my self-imposed deadline.

The day before we told the team, I went running around all over town and calling some friends on the phone, people I wanted to tell before it got out through the media or word of mouth from others.

Telling everyone that I had Parkinson's lifted the weight of the world off my shoulders. I did not have to hide my medication bottles anymore. I didn't have to worry about people noticing those little physical changes that I was experiencing and finding out that way.

I quickly found out how supportive everyone was.

NHL Commissioner Gary Bettman called me. I had never spoken to him before, so it was nice to hear from him.

Cam called me and told me he was sorry to hear and told me that if I had a good attitude like Michael, I would be fine.

We had the lockout the year after I told the team, and after the lockout year, the players sort of forgot about the Parkinson's and just treated me normally. Everybody was great. That was exactly what I needed. When I was at the rink, all I had to do was concentrate on doing my job. I was a much better coach from that point on since I didn't have to worry about keeping the secret as I had done the previous season.

Chapter Four - My Start in the NHL

I was born and raised in Calgary, Alberta. We were an athletic family. I was the oldest of four boys born to my parents Ron and Nurae. I began playing hockey at a nearby rink when I was five-years-old. This was followed by many years of early morning games where my devoted mother would drive me back and forth to and from the rink every day.

I was the starting quarterback on the varsity football team in high school, my twin brothers Doug and Darren played football and basketball in high school, and my other brother Greg went to Brigham Young University on a scholarship and ended up playing professional football in Canada.

Hockey was not in the schools when I was growing up, it was in the community. You played for your city or town's team, not what school you attended.

Basketball and football were in the schools. In Canada, you had the choice between playing major junior hockey or staying in Tier 2 and then going to a Division 1 college hockey school in the United States. Back then, most of the top players in Canada went to junior.

In Calgary, Mike Rogers, Danny Gare, and John Davidson played for the Calgary Centennials from 1971-1973. I grew up loving those guys. John Davidson was a hero of mine. The players on that team were 18-years-old. I was about 14 or 15 going to those games. They never had a pro team in Calgary until then, so I just watched junior hockey.

When I was 14, I belonged to the Calgary Centennials. My dad Ron was a lawyer, so people knew that education was important to him. Thinking that I was going to go to the US, Calgary dropped me off their list. After they dropped me, Edmonton added me to their list, and then the Edmonton people asked me if I would come up and play as a 16-year-old.

I said, "Yeah, I want to be an NHL player, so I have to go."

In high school, I was a good football player. Since I was the quarterback for the football team, everybody was upset with me because I went away to play hockey. I only played Grade 10 as the starting quarterback though. I knew that I wasn't going to make it in football. I was too small and too slow. My future was in hockey.

My mom didn't want me to go because Edmonton was three hours north of Calgary and I had to live with a billet family. I went anyway, and thankfully it worked out well. There were some other good young players on that team like

Paul Mulvey and Wayne Babych.

I played two years in Edmonton with the Oil Kings and then the team moved to Portland, Oregon and became the Portland Winter Hawks. I was named captain of the team when I was 18 and played two years in Portland.

It was tough because a lot of the players were homesick. A lot of the guys were from Edmonton, and because Edmonton was a hotbed of talent, they played right there at home with the Oil Kings.

When Wayne Gretzky came to the Oilers, they moved the junior team down to Portland. That was a thousand miles from Edmonton. I had already been living away from home for two years, so I was fine with it.

At the start, it was hard in Portland. We didn't have any fans for a while, but we had such a good team that year. It was 76-77, and we had a good squad too. One time our coach Ken Hodge came into the locker room before the game.

He told all of our tough guys that they were starting the game. And then he said, "Peterson, you and Babych are up to kill the penalty," because he knew we were going to kill a penalty right off the hop.

Portland was also where I met Tami. She was a senior in high school and I had graduated a year earlier. We had a young team in Portland, so I was a year older than all of the guys on the team, so most of them were still in high school and I was taking classes at a community college. Thanks to a couple of my teammates who were still in high school, I got the opportunity to meet Tami.

So Mulvey and Perry Turnbull saw this cute girl in school one day and tried to chat her up a little. She shot them down pretty much immediately by telling them that she was a Mormon and didn't smoke or drink or anything like that.

As many probably already know, everyone in hockey has at least one nickname. In fact, some guys may not actually know what some of their teammates' real names actually are. Quite often, a player's nickname is a derivative of the first syllable of their last name – case in point, just about everyone calls me Petey.

Of course, being the ball-busting teammates that they were, they told her that I was a bad Mormon; that I smoke, drank, basically all of the things that I was not supposed to do. When they told me that they had met this really pretty Mormon girl, they told me that her family was not a very good Mormon family, but that they just told everyone in town that they were.

One time we were at a football game and she came up to me and she said, "How come you are a bad Mormon?"

I said, "I am not. I am a good guy. I don't drink. I don't smoke. I don't do any of that stuff. Why are your family members not good Mormons?"

"They are," she shot back.

It didn't take us very long to figure out that my teammates were trying to pull one over on us. Well, I should probably say that it didn't take me very long, Tami had not been around hockey players, so she wasn't aware of how we occasionally did things like that to each other.

She had a boyfriend back then, but I used to go over to her house and hang out with her mom because her mom really liked me. Tami would be out on a date with another guy and I would be back at her house. Her mom would even pull her car out of the garage so that I could park mine in there so Tami's boyfriend would not know I was there.

Chapter Five - The Detroit Years

After getting drafted by the Red Wings in 1978, I made the team in training camp that fall. The joy of making the team was quickly replaced by pain and suffering when I broke my right leg in the team's fifth game of the season at the old Detroit Olympia. It was bad; a spiral fracture and both the tibia and fibula were broken. I thought I would be back in three months, but it just didn't heal.

My season was over just after it started. This is not the way you want your NHL career to begin.

I couldn't do much of anything because I had a full length cast on my leg for six months. I was living by myself in a two-story house in Dearborn, Michigan. I had to go up and down stairs on crutches with my leg in this giant cast. I must have fallen ten times with this cast on; down the stairs, in the snow, everywhere you could imagine and even in some you could not imagine.

Obviously I didn't want to go out every night since it was hard to get in and out of the car. And once I got in the car, driving was not easy, and now that I think about it, it probably was not all that safe either. I had to drive using my left foot on the accelerator and the brake. While I was doing this, my right leg was spread over the center console toward the other side of the car.

Since I didn't cook and I had to be on crutches for months, I just called the nearest pizza place that I could find. The only place that I could find that would deliver was Domino's Pizza. Domino's Pizza just happened to start about that time in Ann Arbor, Michigan. The guy would come in the house, put the pizza down on the table, and go get me a glass of milk or something. He would take the money for the pizza and say, "I'll see you tomorrow night." I did that almost every night for five months.

When I played, I played at 195 pounds. With the lack of activity and the less than ideal nutritional program I put myself on, I knew that I had put on a few pounds. Right before I was about to get the cast off in April, I went down to the training room at the Olympia and weighed myself. I could not believe it. When I stepped on the scale, it said I was 225 pounds. Those old plaster casts were heavy, so I thought the cast had to be responsible for a lot of the weight gain, maybe 15 pounds or so.

I went to the doctor and got the cast off and then immediately went back to the dressing room at the Olympia to weigh myself again. The verdict? 223 pounds. That heavy plaster cast only weighed two pounds. I had gained 28 pounds in six months. I had never weighed that much.

By the time I got out of the cast, my leg had atrophied so much; I couldn't even push the accelerator down on the car when I got out of the cast. It is a good thing I had so much experience driving with my left leg or else I would have had a real problem.

Being a professional athlete and being that out of shape was not a good combination. I had a bigger and more immediate problem on my hands though. Tami and I were getting married that summer.

We dated for a year and a half, and I ended up going to Detroit, and she went away to go to school at BYU Idaho. She didn't like going to school there and we missed each other, so we got married the next summer.

Tami was away at school that year, so she had not seen me during my broken leg and pizza-induced weight gain phase. Needless to say, she was shocked when she saw me for the first time. The horror in her eyes showed the fear she had of having a giant husband standing next to her in the wedding photos that we would be looking at for the rest of our lives.

I had to eat a lot of salads, do a lot of running, but I got a lot of the weight off before the wedding that summer, and thankfully Tami married me as scheduled. We were married in the L.D.S. Temple in Cardston, Alberta. Following the wedding, I was able to get the remainder of the extra pounds off and got down to 195 by the next fall's training camp.

We were young. Tami was 21 and I was 22 when our first child, Ryan, was born. We have been together a pretty long time.

Back then; players did not make a lot of money. Nowadays, it is a completely different story with what they earn. Back when I was playing, every time we would go on a road trip, something would break. The washer would break, the garage door would break, or the kids would get sick. Now, Tami fends for herself and she doesn't want me around because I get in the way of her routine. For years, she hadn't even been east of Salt Lake City. She grew up in Portland and she hadn't been anywhere until we got married. She learned from all the wives what to do and what not to do. Now she is a pretty outspoken person. She is pretty confident in her abilities to talk and do things.

In my second season in the NHL, I once again made the team in training camp, but once again I suffered a broken leg. This time I broke the left leg. Fortunately for me, this break was not nearly as severe as the first one. They did not even put a cast on the leg the second time and I was back playing in two months.

One of my teammates in Detroit was Paul Woods, who now does the radio broadcasts for the Red Wings. During our playing days, we were good friends.

We both liked to joke around and one of his favorite things to do was call Tami and conduct fake interviews with her.

When I was away, he would call the house and when she picked up, he would ask for Mrs. Peterson. He knew she was Mrs. Peterson, but he asked anyway.

"This is WK whatever radio in Detroit," he would tell her. "We want to interview you because your husband plays for the Detroit Red Wings."

He would talk to her and conduct what Tami thought was a real interview. He would conclude the interviews by saying, "Thank you very much Mrs. Peterson, we will talk to you later."

Paul would not tell her that it was all a joke. Tami was so young at the time and she was not all that familiar with hockey players and their warped senses of humor. She later found out that it was Paul and she was not happy about it.

Now from time to time actual media outlets would call the house looking to talk to me or talk to Tami if something happened like when I got traded. To this day, there is never a time that she does not think back to the calls Paul made to her 30 years ago. Right after she found out, she was tempted to tell off anyone that called thinking it was Paul. She resisted that urge on the chance that whomever she was talking to happened to be legitimate. Tami did not want to be known as the crazy hockey wife who went off on some poor unsuspecting radio host just looking for a quote from a woman whose husband just got traded.

The pranks were not limited to just Paul prank calling Tami though. And there is a chance that I may have been in on some of those pranks as well.

One cold winter day, Paul and I took the doors off of Dennis Polonich's Jeep Wrangler. We put the doors in the trunk of my car and left. His drive home took about 30 minutes, and he had to do it in the middle of winter with no doors on his Jeep. He was fine though. Hockey players are tough.

Another time, when I wasn't involved, Pete Mahovlich took a big spike and nailed Perry Miller's cowboy boots right into the floor. Perry found out who had done it, so he had to strike back. Pete wore this big cowboy hat to practice the next day. He put it up on the shelf in the locker room. Perry came into the locker room, defecated into the hat, and put it back up on the shelf. Pete was really surprised when he put his hat on after practice that day.

My time in Detroit came to an end in 1981 when I was traded to Buffalo along with Dale McCourt and Mike Foligno in exchange for Derek Smith, Danny Gare, and Jim Schoenfeld. I was considered the throw-in in that deal just so there were not too many guys going to Detroit compared with the number going to Buffalo. Detroit needed something to get them going, and the Sabres had a bunch of veterans, so Scotty Bowman was ready to get all of those veterans out of Buffalo.

Chapter Six - Centering Mr. Hockey

My first introduction to Gordie Howe came in a game played in Springfield, Massachusetts. While I was rehabilitating from a broken leg, I had been playing for the Adirondack Red Wings, but I was called up to Detroit and our next game was on the road against the Hartford Whalers.

That game did not end up being played in Hartford though. After a heavy snowstorm, the Hartford Civic Center's roof collapsed. Thankfully there was no one in the building when that happened so no one was hurt. The game was moved to Springfield, Massachusetts, which is only about 25 miles from Hartford.

When I got called up, Detroit did not have a helmet big enough to fit me. Now my wife disagrees with me on this point, but I do not have that big of a head. Adirondack is located in Glens Falls, New York, and is about a two-hour drive from Springfield, so Tami was nice enough to make the trip to bring me the helmet I had been using in Adirondack. She made the trip by herself and she was four months pregnant with Ryan, our first child, at the time, so it was an impressive effort on her part for sure. Now I will admit that her having to bring me a helmet because the team did not have one big enough to fit me makes it look like she was probably on the winning end of the whether or not I have a big head debate.

Tami had never seen an NHL game before, so she stayed to watch that night's contest. She had also grown up in Portland, Oregon, which is not exactly a hockey town, so she did not really know much about the game or the people who played it... other than me of course.

Since I had just been called up, I was playing on Detroit's fourth line. Gordie was playing on Hartford's fourth line at the time, so we ended up playing against each other all night.

She came up to me after the game, and the first thing she asked me was why they let an old gray-haired man out onto the ice to play in the game. She was scared that someone was going to hurt this old man.

I said to her: "Dear, that's Gordie Howe!"

Her response: "Who is he?"

Then we had a little discussion about exactly who Gordie Howe was.

Eventually, it all came circling back. I ended up playing in Hartford at the end of my career. Gordie was still there as a community services representative for the team. Gordie and I ended up going out to visit all the kids at schools to do the anti-drug talks.

Every year, the Whalers hosted a charity event called the Whalers Waltz. One year Tami and I saw Gordie sitting there, so we went up to him and I told him that I had a funny story to tell him about my wife. While Tami became increasingly more mortified by the minute, I went into great detail in telling him the story about Tami not knowing who he was ten or eleven years earlier. Over the years she learned a lot about the game and the players who played it, but that story was too good not to tell Gordie. He got a great laugh out of it.

After my last year playing, I went into coaching, so then I was on the Whalers' alumni team. Gordie was also on the Whalers' alumni team, and because he was there, we sold out everywhere we played around the New England area. We played against several other alumni teams like ones from the Boston Bruins and the New York Rangers. We had some big crowds, all because Gordie was there. We usually played on a line together. I played center and Gordie would be my right wing.

Gordie used to be the toughest guy ever to play. If a player gets a goal, assist, and a fighting major in a game it is called a Gordie Howe Hat Trick.

In one alumni game, this younger player was running around on the ice. Yes, he was running around during an alumni game. At one point, he ran Gordie's son Marty. After that hit, Gordie went out and said, "Hey kid, calm down."

This kid didn't listen. It was a big mistake, and Gordie had enough of this kid.

So the guy I was set to replace on a change was coming off the ice, and I was going to jump out there.

Gordie said to me, "Just stay there Petey."

Unlike the kid, I listened to Gordie and stayed on the bench so he could take my shift. He jumped over the boards and went down into the corner. He threw a couple elbows and ended up breaking the guy's nose. They had to carry him off of the ice.

Still the tough guy, Gordie said, "I told you to calm down."

Just to remind you, this was an alumni game being played for charity, but he was warned. The guy had to get stitches, but he should have known better than to ignore a warning from Gordie Howe. He may have been 63-years-old at the time, but Gordie only knew how to play the game one way. He is one of the nicest people in the world too, but he is also about the toughest person in the world as well and not someone whose bad side you want to be on if you do not want to end up getting stitches.

I have a picture of Gordie hanging in my office. The picture says, "To Brent from your right winger," and signed Gordie Howe. Looking at that picture every day is something that is really special to me.

When Gordie turned 80 in 2008, the Predators were playing in Detroit the night the Red Wings celebrated his birthday with a ceremony before the game. The way the schedule turned out, we just happened to be there that night, and it was a great honor to be there for that experience and witness how the Detroit organization and their fans paid tribute to the man known to most as Mr. Hockey. A lot of people can call him Mr. Hockey, but very few can call him a linemate.

Chapter Seven - Adventures with Scotty

After I was traded to Buffalo, I did not play much at the start. We went through that year and I played a little bit at the end of the season. Craig Ramsay was on my line for the next two or three years, or I was on his line I guess I should say. This is when I learned all about hockey.

Craig taught me all about penalty killing and about defensive play. I had already experienced two broken legs, so I had to find a niche. I was a scorer in junior, but I slowed down because of the injuries. I learned how to check, I learned how to take faceoffs, and I learned how to kill penalties. Without doing those kinds of things, there was no way I was going to be able to stay in the league.

Rammer had eight twenty-goal seasons over the course of his career. In 1985, he won the Selke Trophy as the league's top defensive forward. I finished high in the Selke voting that season as well. We were number one in penalty killing three of the four years I was in Buffalo. I was one of the top faceoff guys all those years too.

Scotty Bowman was the general manager of the Sabres. He came in and out of coaching the team for several years. Scotty was old school. He didn't want to try to get close to his players because he knew he had to cut them or trade them at some point. He was a tough guy, but he was very fair to me and very generous to me in my contracts and with my playing time. He knew what I did for the team and he respected me for my contributions.

Whether or not it was intentional, and sometimes it wasn't, Scotty was funny.

When we played for Scotty, he had a strict rule that nobody would go over the bench until we were told to do so because he wanted to match lines.

Sometimes his line change calls came very late though, so it got confusing on the bench. One game later on in my Buffalo career, the other team was regrouping in their end, so four or five of our guys all came over to the bench for a change. This happened to be one of the times where Scotty had failed to tell us who was up next.

We were very disciplined, but we were yelling, "Who is up?" Then he panicked and started screaming, "Jump, jump, somebody jump. Who do you guys think I am Van Halen? Jump. Anybody jump."

This happened not too long after Van Halen's song "Jump" was released, so among all the chaos of trying to figure out who was going on the ice, hearing our coach asking if we thought he was Van Halen was unbelievably funny.

There was no telling how many guys came over the bench at that point, but one thing is for sure was that they were all laughing as they did.

The 1982-83 season was my best. As far as my offensive production was concerned, I had 13 goals, 24 assists, and 37 points; all career highs. We were first in penalty killing, I was one of the top faceoff guys, and I had all these stats. I did my own contract with Scotty since I decided that I didn't need an agent because I wasn't going to make a lot of money. I was just an average player.

We lived in Portland in the summer because that is where Tami is from. Scotty was in Portland that offseason because the Memorial Cup was being played there and he was there scouting that tournament.

"Scotty can I meet with you about my contract," I asked him.

"Yeah, but I don't know why," he responded.

He liked to talk in circles. He was always talking about one thing and then he would just change the subject without any warning.

So I met up with him and I was giving him my rundown with all of my stats.

"You are my fourth line centerman. You can't skate. You can't score. I called Jersey and even Jersey doesn't want you," he said in a very matter of fact manner.

"What are we talking about this kind of money for?"

I think I was making $100,000 at the time on a one-way contract. Then he just jumped to asking me about living in Portland and what it was like. It was a quick transition from telling me that I couldn't play to asking me about Portland, but I rolled with him and his odd conversational pattern.

"Yeah Scotty," I said. "It is a nice place to live."

"It rains too much for me," he proclaimed.

Then he quickly switched back to the contract discussion, albeit briefly.

"Ahh... I don't want to talk about this anymore. Just fax me what kind of money you think you should make."

At this point my head was spinning. How could it not be with that kind of interaction?

So I called my friend Ed Chynoweth who was president of the Western Hockey League and I told him that he had to help me with this contract. I asked Scotty for $110,000, $120,000, and $130,000 for three years, just a $10,000 increase each year. I didn't ask for any bonuses because I wasn't going to score any goals. All I wanted was a one-way contract.

Two weeks later, I got a call from Ed. He asked if I had sent something different to Scotty.

"He must have thought you were a different guy because he came back and offered you a contract of $130,000, $140,000, and $150,000," Ed said.

Scotty gave me more than I had asked for plus he gave me an additional $1,000 retroactive for each year because I was in the best shape in camp.

I told Ed I didn't know what Scotty was doing, but I wanted to sign it quickly before he changed his mind or figured out he sent the offer to the wrong player.

At training camp that fall, it took Scotty all of one day to get on Mike Ramsey, Larry Playfair, and me.

"Peterson, Playfair, Ramsey, did I treat you guys well this summer?" Scotty yelled.

"Yes Scotty."

He pointed at Larry and said, "You guys like this guy?"

Larry was a really popular player, so everybody said yes.

"You really like him? Because he is really in trouble, he is really struggling," Scotty said. "This is the first day of camp. You guys better wake up. We had a terrible scrimmage. I took care of him this summer and you better be careful or else he is going to be gone."

One game in Buffalo against Washington, Scotty somehow lost track of the score of the game.

We were up 2-0, and at the end of the second period, we gave up a goal. Scotty came in the locker room and was screaming at us. In his mind, we were tied, but we were really up by a goal.

"The way you played that period, you are lucky we are still tied," he said.

One of our guys went out to check the scoreboard after Scotty's rant, and sure enough we were up 2-1 like everyone thought, save for Scotty, though.

So we went out for the third period and they scored a goal. Now it was tied, but in Scotty's mind we were down by one. He was looking at the clock the whole time, and for some reason he couldn't see what the score was.

In the last minute, our guys were coming off for a change, so Scotty was set to put the offensive guys out next. Our goalie was Bobby Sauve, and Scotty was waiving for him to come to the bench for the extra attacker. Despite our best efforts to tell Scotty that the game was tied, it did not work.

Right then the Capitals took a penalty. At this point, Scotty was all confused and did not know who to put on the ice. For some reason he put my line out on the power play, and I think he realized what he did after sending us out, but it was too late to make a change. We were a shutdown and penalty-killing group, so this power play time was new to us.

Guys like Mike Ramsey, Craig Ramsay, Billy Hajt, and I were all out there. Mike Ramsey had never been on the power play before. Craig had probably never been on many power plays either.

Right before the faceoff, I said to Rammer, "What do we do?"

"If you win the draw, go to the front of the net," he said.

So I won the draw to Mike Ramsey, he threw it to Billy Hajt, back to Mike Ramsey, and Mike Ramsey threw it on net. In what can only be described as a hockey miracle, the puck went off of my ass and into the net. That was the game-winning goal.

Scotty was the hero because he had the right guys on the ice and all because he didn't know the score. After the game when the reporters were asking Scotty about his curious choice of players for a late-game power play, he played it cool and told them he just had a feeling about Peterson's line.

A few of the guys in Detroit told me that Scotty always used to talk to his team through Barry Smith, who was his assistant for many years in both Pittsburgh and Detroit. Scotty was a brilliant coach, a brilliant tactician, and brilliant behind the bench. He loved the game, studied the game, and was always up to date on anything. Scotty was talking to the team, but he was talking through Smitty.

"They don't listen to me, nobody listens to me," Scotty would say.

The play would be going on and the players would ask Scotty who is up? He would say, "I don't care, you guys don't listen to me."

That's why they always had guys all over the place just jumping over the boards going to all positions. One time play was going on and he noticed that someone was sitting in his seats in the stands.

"Smitty," he said. "Somebody is sitting in my seats. I didn't give away my tickets tonight. Who is in my seats? Go find out who is in my seats."

This is all while the play was going on. The guys were just laughing on the bench.

One time when the Predators were playing in Joe Louis Arena, Mitch Korn, our goaltending coach, had his father with him. Everyone called Mitch's father Pop Korn. Pop Korn had a little bit of dementia. Mitch had to go out onto the ice for practice, and he asked me to watch his dad for 15 minutes. So his dad walked out of the room toward the Zamboni tunnel. I lost sight of him and came barreling out of the room to go get him. As I turned the corner Scotty was right in my face.

"What are you doing?" he said.

"I am following Pop Korn around," I said while trying to keep an eye on Pop Korn.

"Well who is that?"

"It's Mitch Korn's father Scotty," I said.

"Well what is he doing?"

He asked me about 40 questions in about two minutes. I told Scotty that Pop Korn had a little bit of dementia, and that Mitch had asked me to follow him around.

"What are you going to do with him?" Scotty asked.

Before I could even generate an answer to that question he shifted gears again.

"We don't score enough goals in this league," he said. "We need bigger nets."

"I gotta go Scotty," I said trying to get away. "I need to follow Pop Korn around."

"We gotta score more," he said as I was finally able to break away from him.

Scotty motivated in different ways. He also knew how to handle players. In Detroit, he took care of the stars and made sure they were on his side. He made them better players. They had to play a little bit of defense and they led the way. Steve Yzerman went from being a good captain to a great captain and Scotty was the reason for that. He is a funny and interesting guy. I wasn't scared of him, but I was a little intimidated by him.

In 2008, the draft was in Ottawa. We stayed downtown and had to make the long drive to the Senators' arena, which is in Kanata. The bus from the draft would come and pick us up first at our hotel before it made the rest of the stops. Trotzy, some of the other guys, and I were about the only ones to get on when we left because the scouts all went early. We were getting there just in time for the draft.

At the next stop, Ken Holland, Scotty, and all of the Detroit people got on the bus. At that point, there were only about four seats taken on the bus and we were spread out around the bus. The Detroit guys got on the bus, and even though they had the whole bus to choose from, Scotty came and sat down right beside me. For an hour, he was engaging and was great to talk to. Sometimes when you played for Scotty, he wouldn't know you were in the same hallway. This day, he was asking me all kinds of questions and we had a great conversation.

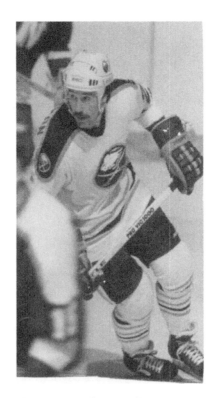

Brent as a Sabre (Buffalo Sabres)

Chapter Eight - An Early Start to my Coaching Career

When I was playing in Buffalo, Scotty was ready to pass Dick Irvin on the all time list for wins as a coach. We went about three games without winning, and he was getting pretty frustrated. He had never picked on me before, but he had always picked on the other guys. We were going to Chicago to play the Blackhawks. Denis Savard was their big star at the time.

Scotty called me into his office the day before we were leaving for Chicago. I always got the assignment to cover the other team's top player.

"Where are we going tomorrow?" Scotty asked.

"Chicago," I said, wondering where the conversation was going.

"You can't keep up to Savard," he said dealing a serious blow to my ego. "You aren't good enough. I called Jersey and even Jersey doesn't want you."

Now this is the second time in my years of playing for Buffalo that Scotty had told me that he had called Jersey and they didn't want me. Did he say that to all of the players as a motivational tool, or did he just really want me gone so badly that he called everyone including the Devils trying to get rid of me?

"Just go home and we will call you," he said. "You aren't going with the team."

I was a regular player, the number one faceoff guy, and played a lot. All of a sudden I was not even in the lineup or even going on the road with the team.

My mom just happened to be in town and I was out playing street hockey with the kids. Later that afternoon the phone rang.

"Brent, it is Scotty Bowman," my mom yelled from the house.

As I am heading into the house to take the call, I am thinking, "I am traded. He has traded me already. Am I going to Jersey?"

"Hello?" I said.

"It's Scotty," the voice on the other end of the phone said. "I want you to be at the plane tomorrow morning."

Back then, on our short trips to Chicago and other places that were not that far away, we used to fly in the morning, eat our pregame meal, lay down for a nap in the afternoon, play the game in the evening, and then fly home after the game so we didn't have to stay overnight. We had a 10:00 flight going to Chicago, and we gained an hour with the time change, so we got in there about 11:30-12:00.

The equipment guy, Rip Simonick, saw me at the airport and approached me.

"Petey, what are you doing here?" he asked. "Scotty told me not to bring your equipment."

"I don't know what I am doing," I told him. "He just told me to be here."

So I had none of my equipment with me, and I am going to Chicago. So I went and found our assistant coach Joe Crozier.

"He hasn't said a word to me," Joe said.

I went and had the pregame meal, had a nap, and then later went down to the bus. We had a meeting at 5:30 for the 7:00 game.

I saw Joe before the meeting and asked him again what going on.

"I have no idea Brent," he responded. "I haven't talked to him."

After the meeting, I saw Joe. He handed me a walkie-talkie and told me to take the walkie-talkie and go up to the top of the arena to talk to him on the walkie-talkie while he was on the bench.

In Chicago Stadium there were separate stairs in each corner going up to different press boxes. You couldn't get from one to the other because they were separated. I went all the way to the top, and it turned out that I was in the wrong press box.

So I went all of the way back down and then went all the way up to the right press box. When I heard the National Anthem starting, I looked down at the bench and Joe Crosier was waving and pointing at the walkie-talkie. I turned it on and he said, "I messed up. I am supposed to be up there and you are supposed to be down here on the bench."

I went all the way down the stairs, and Joe came off of the ice. I had to wait because in the old Chicago Stadium, you had to stand there and wait because you had to go across the ice to get to the benches. I waited about four minutes for the play to stop. Once play came to a halt, I trotted across the ice.

The players were asking me what was going on. Joe had gone off the ice and up to the top, and when I hopped over the bench, Scotty said, "Cheer loud."

I went behind the bench. I was all active and everything just like what I thought an assistant coach would do, and we won the game 7-3. Scotty broke Dick Irvin's record with that win.

Following the Chicago game, we went to Quebec City. The Quebec Nordiques usually killed us. Our centermen were Gilbert Perreault, John Tucker, Dave Andreychuk, and me. They had Stastny, Hunter, and Andre Savard. I was back behind the bench because we won with me there the game before. We were beaten 5-1 in that game. It was Thursday night in Chicago, Saturday night in Quebec, and then back at home Sunday night.

After we got beaten in Quebec, Scotty called a meeting at the practice rink in the morning. I hadn't skated in like four days. After the meeting, he called in Andreychuk, Tucker, Perreault, and me for a talk. Joe Crozier was there because he had been there for all the different meetings. Joe was sitting there quietly.

Scotty turned to Perreault and said, "Gilbert, you just do your own thing. You can leave."

Andreychuk and Tucker were like 19-20 years old, and they didn't know what was going on at that point.

Scotty said, "John, on a scale of one to five, what would you rate yourself last night?"

"I was probably a two," John said.

Scotty pointed at him and said, "You were a minus one."

And just to be clear, Scotty was not talking about his plus/minus rating.

Then he pointed at Andreychuk. Andreychuk was a happy go lucky guy, and he didn't know what to say.

"I was probably a one or a two," Andy said.

"You were a minus three," Scotty shot back.

Again, he was not talking about Andreychuk's plus/minus.

After that, Scotty went into this long lecture. Joe Crosier was over in the corner snickering the whole time.

"Peterson is the only one I can rely on," Scotty announced to the group. "He wins faceoffs and he checks the other team's top players."

He went on and on after that. Scotty played me that night, and I think he played me about 40 minutes. I couldn't get off the ice. So I was back in the lineup again after that.

I went from being a regular player, to being a bum, to an assistant coach, and back to playing all in the span of about four days.

Maybe the two-game stint as an assistant was a result of Scotty seeing some potential in me as a coach, but I was thankful that it was over quickly and I was back to being a player.

That was Scotty. As a player, you never really knew what was going on inside his head. I think he liked it that way. Looking at his record, no one can really argue with the results and all of those Stanley Cup victories.

Chapter Nine - Checking the Great One

As the center of the checking line for the teams that I played for through the years, one of the assignments I always drew was playing against Wayne Gretzky's line when we were up against the Edmonton Oilers. Now measuring success against Gretzky is relative, but I did a pretty decent job of trying to keep him somewhat in check in the games I played against him. Of course, he won four more Stanley Cups and nine more Hart Trophies than I did, so pretty much no one shut him down during his amazing career.

One game in Edmonton, we played great all night against Gretzky. It was 2-2 into the third period.

Before the game, we had a talk about their goaltender Grant Fuhr. Someone said, "If you deke him when you get in alone with him, he will spread his legs, so you can make one move and throw it five hole."

They were the run and gun team of the 80s. They made wild passes all over the ice. They were a great team, but we did a great job on Gretzky and Mark Messier that night. With about 20 seconds to go in the third, someone tried to throw a cross-ice pass. I intercepted the puck just outside the Edmonton blue line, and I went in from the blue line all alone on Fuhr.

So I was thinking back to the conversation we had before the game, and when I got in on Fuhr, I pulled him and tried to put it between his legs. Of course things did not work out exactly as they were planned. Fuhr stopped the shot I attempted to put between his pads, it went in the corner, and the horn blew. This was before the NHL instituted overtime. Game over. 2-2.

Scotty came into the locker room and we could tell that he was a little bit mad.

"Peterson, you aren't good enough to make that move," he said. "You have to pick a spot and shoot it."

Jimmy Matheson, who is one of the Edmonton beat writers, came in the locker room and asked me what I was thinking on the breakaway. I have known Jimmy for years, so as usual, I had a little fun at my own expense.

"I went in like Wayne Gretzky and I came out like Brent Peterson," I told him.

That was my quote in the paper the next day. I am still pretty proud of that one.

Part of the reason for my success in checking Gretzky all those years was my ability to, let's say, bend the rules a little bit. We used to grab sticks, hook, hold, and do pretty much everything we could possibly get away with in an attempt to slow him down. We got away with murder back then. The referees never called anything, and this was back in the day when there was only one referee on the ice. Now there are two referees on the ice and they are calling a much tighter game than when I played.

During most of his playing days, Gretzky used Titan hockey sticks. A lot of the top players used Titans, but Gretzky made them famous. He usually used the red sticks with the white writing.

One game we were playing Edmonton in Buffalo. I think it was 3-3 for just about the whole game. I was playing center. I beat Gretzky on draws most of the time because that is about all I could do. Because he was such a great player, I would grab his stick the whole time. He got a little bit ticked off and he became worse as we got toward the end of the game.

At the end of the game, he skated up to me and said, "You know what Brent, if you like my sticks that much, I can get a dozen of them for you if you want."

Years later, Gretzky was in charge of Hockey Canada. At the 2001 World Championships in Germany, Wayne Fleming was the head coach and Guy Carbonneau and I were the assistant coaches. Trotzy couldn't go, so they made me one of the assistant coaches. Lanny McDonald and Steve Tambellini were all there with Hockey Canada as well. We were in Hanover.

One of my jobs was to skate all of the guys who were extras. Gretzky was back at the hotel with the guys that were going to play. Later Wayne came up to me and asked if he could come skate with us. He just wanted to go for a whirl, and what was I going to say to Wayne Gretzky, no?

Tambellini then said he wanted to go out on the ice, then Lanny McDonald and Guy Carbonneau and so on, so it was turning into a pretty good group. We had some of the top players ever to play the game out on the ice that day. So we picked teams, and it just so happened that Gretzky, Tambellini, and McDonald all got put together on the same team. They were all stars and the big scorers of their day. Carbonneau and I, and all the checkers were on the other side. Carbonneau was a checker and I was a checker, so Gretzky looked across the ice and said, "I have to play against you guys again?"

One of the janitors saw Gretzky. A couple of players from teams from other countries were there too. Word started to spread around Hanover pretty quickly, and before too long, we had hundreds of people watching us play a pick-up 3-on-3 game because Wayne Gretzky was on the ice. It was a pretty cool thing to be a part of at the time. It had been a long time since that many people watched me play a hockey game.

During the game, I grabbed Gretzky's stick one time. He turned to me and said,

"You still love those Titans, don't you Petey?"

After all those years, and all of the guys that played against him, he remembered me grabbing his sticks during all of those games we played against each other. Come to think of it, I never did get one of those Titans from him. I wonder if he still has any of them lying around the house.

Chapter Ten - Meeting My Idol

Growing up, my favorite player was Bobby Orr. After I made the team in my first season in Detroit, I was looking forward to our sixth game of the season because we were supposed to play the Chicago Blackhawks, and Bobby Orr was playing for Chicago then.

As luck would have it, I broke my leg in our fifth game of the season, so I missed my chance to play against him. Even though I couldn't play in the game, there was no chance I was going to miss seeing Bobby Orr play. When I got out of the hospital, I went right to Olympia Arena. I sat down right in the Zamboni area so I could be as close to the action as I possibly could without actually playing in the game.

In the game, one of our guys went around Bobby Orr. He couldn't turn because his knee was so bad. He retired the next day, so I never had the opportunity to play against him.

Years later, when I was an assistant coach with the Hartford Whalers, I got a chance to meet Bobby.

Eddie Johnston was the general manager of the Whalers then, and he and Bobby became friends when they played together with the Boston Bruins. Bobby was the big star of the team, and of the whole league for that matter, and Eddie was the backup goalie for the Bruins. When Eddie became the GM of the Whalers, he brought Bobby on as a consultant with the team. Bobby lived in Boston, so it was easy for him to get to Hartford for our games.

On game nights, I was the assistant coach who went upstairs and talked to the bench on the radio. The first night Bobby was there, I went upstairs and he was sitting in the seat right next to me. I couldn't believe it.

The first thing I did was call Tami. I was whispering into the phone so that he wouldn't hear me. Of course since I was whispering, Tami could not hear me very well either. I must have sounded like a two-year-old whispering into the phone gushing over Bobby Orr sitting next to me, but I didn't really care. Each game that he came to in Hartford he sat in the seat right next to me.

Meeting him was great. He is one of the nicest people I have ever met. Bobby is a first-class person. Being a great hockey player is one thing, but it really says something about a guy when someone you looked up to as a kid turns out to be such a good person.

Hartford was not the only place I got to work with Bobby either. My last year coaching the Portland Winter Hawks, we had the best record in the Western Hockey League, so I was given the opportunity to coach one of the teams in the Canadian Hockey League's Top Prospects Game in Toronto.

Each year, Bobby and Don Cherry each have a team in the game, and I got to coach Team Orr. Brian Kilrea from the Ottawa 67's coached Team Cherry that year. I am proud to say that Bobby and I whipped Don and Brian's butts that year.

I did not ask for it, but after the game there was a picture of Bobby Orr in my office. It was the picture of him flying through the air after scoring the Stanley Cup-winning goal in 1970. On the picture, Bobby wrote, "Brent – Great working with you, Bobby Orr."

There is no question how special of a moment that was for me, and that picture is still one of my prized possessions.

Looking back, I wish that I had the foresight to bring a picture of my most famous goal with me to sign and give to Bobby. Of course, I would need to identify which of my 72 career NHL goals would stand out above the others to earn the honor of being my most famous goal. I never won a Stanley Cup let alone scored the Stanley Cup-winning goal, so Bobby has me on that one. And I have never scored a goal while flying through the air, so again, advantage Bobby.

Ahh who am I kidding? The argument of my most famous goal begins and ends with the power-play goal that went into the net off of my ass. Of course, I do not know if a photo of that goal actually exists or not. The photographers in attendance that night probably saw my line out on the ice and thought that there was no chance anything of substance would happen then, so they probably put their cameras down to take a little break. Little did they know that history was about to be made on that particular shift.

What a picture that would be; a puck deflecting off of the back of my hockey pants. Below it, I would sign, "Bobby – Great working with you, Brent Peterson." Something tells me that Bobby would not cherish that picture of me as much as I cherish that one of him, but maybe once I told him the story about Scotty forgetting the score of that game and putting my line on the ice in the game's last minute, he would have a good story to tell to go along with the picture.

The year I coached in the Top Prospects Game was the year before I came to Nashville. David, Trotzy, and all of the scouts were up in the stands watching the prospects game. It was the year before the Predators came into the league, so all of the people from Nashville were there to watch all of the kids who were playing in the game.

They were watching me too it appears. Craig Channel is a good friend of mine and was Nashville's head scout at the time. He introduced me to David and all of the other guys who were there with the Predators.

Chapter Eleven - From Player to Coach

My last season in Buffalo was 1984-85. The following season I was exposed in the waiver draft and claimed by the Vancouver Canucks. After two seasons in Vancouver, I was exposed in the waiver draft again and claimed by Hartford.

It's funny, in the span of three years I was not good enough to be protected by my team, but another team thought enough of me to claim me number one in the waiver draft on two different occasions. Back then, at the end of the training camp, teams used to protect 16 skaters and two goalies.

After my second year in Hartford, I could not play anymore. I had only played 11 NHL seasons, but my playing days had come to an end.

Eddie Johnston was taking over as general manager in Hartford and he was going to get a new coach. He told me that really liked me and wanted me to interview with Ricky Lee. Ricky interviewed me and hired me. I became the assistant coach for the same team for whom I had played just a year before. That's hard to do and you shouldn't do that, but I did and that is how I got my start in coaching.

I stayed in Hartford for two seasons as assistant coach, and then the Portland Winter Hawks of the Western Hockey League came calling. The general manager and coach wanted to retire from coaching, and he called me asking me if I was interested. I thought it was a great opportunity to go back to the team that I played for in my junior years, not to mention the fact that it was Tami's hometown, so she was excited to go back. To come back, the team offered me a three percent ownership stake.

I became part owner, director of hockey operations and co-coach of the Winter Hawks. After co-coaching together for two years, I became the head coach and stayed in that position for five more years. Our sons, Ryan and Brad, were with me at the home games and some on the road too.

In my last season in Portland, we won the Memorial Cup. I had Brenden Morrow, Marian Hossa, and Andrew Ference on that team, so it would have been pretty hard for me to screw that team up without trying very hard. We never lost two games in a row that year. We were 53-14-5 during the season. We had a great team.

Portland is where I learned how to coach. I learned how to teach, build relationships with players, and do everything that had to do with coaching.

For people who did not know me back then, this may come as a bit of a surprise, but I was a little more animated on the bench during my head coaching days in Portland. I got into all kinds of trouble with the league because I liked to throw water bottles and rule books at the referees. I was fined all the time, and we didn't make much money there either.

One time, I thought the referee didn't know the rules, so I went in and got a rule book and I threw it on the ice. I said, "Read this, it is a pretty good read." After the game, I got a fine for that.

The fine for throwing a water bottle started at $100, but since I did it so often, I was considered a repeat offender, so each water bottle I threw cost me $200. Imagine going through a coaching career being known as the guy who is a repeat water bottle offender. That was me. Believe it or not, I always waited until the end of the game to throw my water bottles though. Everyone thought I was crazy. I never got kicked off the bench, and I never cost my team a penalty to put us shorthanded.

The last time I was fined was towards the end of the 1997-98 season. I made that one count, because in that game, I threw three water bottles at the referee after the game. My aim was not all that good that night, so when the first two that I threw failed to connect with their intended target, I threw a third.

Rick Doerksen was, and still is for that matter, the Western Hockey League's disciplinarian. Doerky called me after the three water bottle night and told me that since I threw three that I was being fined $600.

Being the joker that I am, I tried to tell him that each of those water bottles was only half-full, so that I really should only be fined $300 for throwing three half-full water bottles. Needless to say, he did not find that anywhere near as amusing as I did.

"I'm not paying," I told him. "Tami won't give me any money, so I am not paying the fine."

Doerky knew Tami, so I thought that would help my cause in getting out of paying money we really didn't have. That didn't work, so I came up with what I thought was a fair way of settling the fine. I told him that I would pay him over the next year, and so each time I saw him, I would hand him a $20 bill. Who knows how much I actually ended up giving him, but I am sure that I did not make it up to the $600 I owed. After that season I left Portland for Nashville.

At the 2011 NHL Entry Draft in Minnesota, I saw Doerky sitting with all of the WHL's general managers. Seeing an opportunity, I walked over toward where they were all sitting and made sure everyone could hear me when I said, "Hey Doerky, I still owe you $20 from that last water bottle I threw in 1998."

Most of those guys knew me and my reputation for throwing water bottles, so everyone up there died laughing. After the laughter died down, Doerky shot back, "I think we can let it go after 13 years. You don't have to pay it."

Not all of my missteps in the WHL came as a result of throwing things though.

One game, we were playing Kamloops and Don Hay was their coach. They were the best team and we were the second best. There were about two minutes to go in the game, and stupidly, I put my best line on the ice. In junior you didn't have a lot of lines. Don put his goon squad over and they jumped all over my guys. I yelled at Don on the other bench and I went on and on calling him every name in the book.

Right after that, he put his tough guys on again, and I banged the glass between the benches and the glass broke. My son Brad was on our bench, he was in high school at the time. After I broke the glass, both benches emptied and it was absolute chaos. I got suspended for a game. Thankfully we won that one without me behind the bench.

My most famous outburst as a junior coach did not involve throwing a rule book or a water bottle though. I really stepped over the line when I threatened to kill a referee.

Hank Aarsen was a referee and he was in Tier 2 most of the time, but he would get called up for some WHL games. One game, we were playing at home on a Wednesday against Seattle. Seattle was a really tough team. We had a lot of guys away at World Juniors, so we were very short on the bench. Before the game, I called Hank over, and I said, "Hank, if we are winning the game by one or two goals, it is going to take 30 minutes to play the last three minutes of the game because they are just going to fight, fight, and fight some more."

So sure enough, we were winning by two goals, and it was fight after fight after fight. So I only had five guys left on the bench at the end of the game. After the game, I went on the ice after Hank. Mike Williamson, my assistant coach, was grabbing me, and I said, "No, I just have to go over and talk to him."

Mike had my arms, and I was screaming at Hank. I said, "Hank, if it is the last thing I do, I am going to follow you to the ends of the Earth and I am going to kill you." And then I went off the ice.

Then Ed Chynoweth, who was the league president, called me and asked me what I said to him.

"I don't remember exactly Ed," I said. "It was an emotional game and things got out of hand there at the end. I think that I may have said something about tracking him down and killing him."

So Ed suspended me for three games for that little episode.

Our team was leaving on Thursday and playing Friday, Saturday, and Sunday with games in Medicine Hat, Calgary, and Lethbridge.

So our general manager told me that since I had nothing to do because of the suspension, he wanted me to go to Powell River, British Columbia to go watch a player on our list that no one had ever seen.

Getting to Powell River is like the movie *Planes Trains and Automobiles*. It is way up past Victoria. Honestly, I had to go on a plane, a boat, and then a bus to get there. So I traveled all day Friday and got there Friday night about 7:25. I walked into the building right before faceoff. Hank Aarsen, who refereed our game Wednesday night in Portland, was refereeing the game Friday night in Powell River.

Now remember, just two days prior, I had told Hank that I was going to track him down and kill him. After the game, I went down to the referee's room and knocked on the door. Hank opened the door, and his face went white when he saw me. I think he may have crapped his pants right there too. Right when he opened the door I said, "I told you I would find you Hank."

So I told him to get his stuff off, and we would go talk. So I talked to him about controlling the game and knowing the situation and knowing what was going on. We have been fine ever since.

I had what I considered to be a Duke or a North Carolina type of job there in Portland, but we had the opportunity in Nashville and we went on blind faith. I could have stayed in Portland forever. It was hard because I was the boss and the head coach with the Winter Hawks. We were drawing 8,000 fans a game. People loved us, but I just decided that I wanted to be in the NHL. I didn't know whether I could do it, but I got into a great situation with David and Barry. We just seemed to fall in love with Nashville.

Tami was from Portland, I was the big coaching star there, but I was ready to leave.

Everyone in Portland was happy for me. They thought anybody could do that job because they were a good organization, but they found out really fast that I was a pretty good coach. What is really neat about Portland is that I can still walk down the streets there and people will recognize me, and I haven't worked there since 1998.

Chapter Twelve - Hey Coach, Can You Grab My Bag?

I had met Trotzy a couple of times before I interviewed with him for the job of assistant coach with the Predators, but to say that I knew him very well would not be accurate. He had been named head coach soon after Nashville had been granted an expansion franchise and spent the year between then and when the team started playing out scouting, so our paths had crossed a couple of times that year while I was coaching Portland and at the All-Star game for the Canadian Hockey League.

Since I started coaching it was my dream to become a head coach in the NHL, so I knew that my best chance of achieving that dream would be to get back to the NHL as an assistant. We had a great team in Portland my final year there, and we made it to and won the Memorial Cup, which is the championship of the CHL. It is a four-team tournament; the winners of the Western, Ontario, and Quebec leagues, plus the team from the host city.

What a lot of people did not know was that I was in agony pretty much my entire final season in Portland due to a ruptured disk in my back. I did not want to leave the team, so I postponed the necessary surgery until after the season was completed.

Two days after winning the Memorial Cup, I had the surgery on my back. The doctors told me that I couldn't travel for two weeks, and I had informed the Predators of this fact since they had expressed interest in interviewing me for an assistant coaching position.

Ten days after the surgery, I boarded a plane in Portland and flew to Nashville to interview with the Predators. In what I thought was a nice touch, Trotzy picked me up at the airport. A lot of people probably don't know this, but Barry always likes to pick guys up at the airport if he can. If we trade for a player and Barry is able to do so, he drives to the airport himself. I don't think that there are a lot, if any, other NHL coaches who would do that for one of their players. It is just the kind of guy Trotzy is.

In dealing with the players, he is tough but fair. The players know that they can always go into his office and talk to him. Sometimes they would have an issue with how much they were playing or what role they were playing and they would want to talk about what was bothering them. They may not have liked what they were told, but Barry always shot straight with them on where they stood. As a player, it may be tough to hear what he has to say, but that level of straightforwardness in a person is something that has to be respected.

After flying across the country for my interview, I was in so much pain, I could not even lift my suitcase off of the conveyor belt at baggage claim, so I went ahead and asked Barry if he could carry the bag for me. Looking back, it is pretty funny that here I am coming to interview for a job with this guy and I had to ask him to carry my bag for me.

Barry, of course, had no problem doing it. That is just the kind of guy he is. He really would do anything he could to help someone. That is an admirable quality in anyone, but especially for a person with such a demanding and stressful job description.

As the years went on and my Parkinson's progressed, on the days I was locked up, I would shuffle my feet as I walked. If we were in the office, Trotzy would hear me coming down the hall. He would yell to me, "Don't you dare come in here and touch me."

He was worried that I was going to come into his office and give him a big shock with all of the static electricity that I had built up from shuffling my feet on the carpet. I am thankful that we had the kind of relationship where we could joke around about things like Parkinson's.

Just inside the main doors to the Predators' front offices at Bridgestone Arena is a picture on the left wall. The picture is Trotzy, Peter, and me staring upward. It looks like we are admiring a beautiful sunset or something, but in reality we are just looking at the scoreboard clock prior to the start of a game.

Before we played a game, I always had a pregame ritual that I felt we needed to do in order to be successful.

I am not superstitious. I just like routine. I drive the same way to the game and like to do the same thing at the same time of the day. When I played, I had a routine. I always dressed from left to right; left shin pad, right shin pad, left elbow pad, right elbow pad, etc. and I always did it at the same time. Then I laced my skates up loosely and after that I would tighten them up, first left then right. I wouldn't call it a ritual, but it was just how I did things.

When I got into coaching, I did meetings at the same time, I drove to work the same way and at the same time, and if the bridge was closed, I was screwed.

Once Trotzy and I started coaching together, he kind of followed along.

We had our assignments before the game. Peter and I would go and get the other team's lineup before the game and then Peter would go into the locker room and put that lineup on the board in the room. I would stay out to make sure that the players got off of the ice because the NHL has a rule that if the players do not get off of the ice within 30 seconds of the clock going to zero in the warmup, it is a $10,000 fine. Some guys would like to stay out there, so I would have to start yelling at them to get off of the ice. After the last player came off, I would follow him down the tunnel and then throw my gum out in a certain trashcan down the hall on the way to the coaches room.

I always had to have Big Red gum, but I changed it up my last year of coaching. I would put it in before warmup, chew it during warmup, and throw it out after the warmup.

One time, Brad and some of the trainers had a little fun with me by hiding the trashcan on me. So as I came down the hall, I started to throw my gum in the trashcan, but it was not there. I had nowhere to go with my gum and must have looked really puzzled. They were all standing behind the door laughing at me. They messed around with my routine.

Some nights Trotzy would need a hand getting his suit jacket on, and the last few years, I needed help getting my jacket on as well. It was just something we did for each other.

With 10:00 to go on the clock, I would chew another piece of Big Red gum. We would always come down the tunnel and at 1:58 on the clock, I would throw my gum out in the tunnel underneath the stands. At 1:54 we would step onto the bench; Trotzy would go first, I would go second, and Peter would be third. We did that every period. If we got on a losing streak, we would try to change things up a little, but the clock would always have to be on a four for some reason; 2:04, 2:14, something different, but still on a four. When we were in buildings like San Jose were we had to walk across the ice to get to the bench, we would go at 3:04 to give ourselves an extra minute to get there. We were pretty funny.

On the road it is hard to get in too many routines because all of the buildings are a little different, but one thing we could control was what time we got on the bench. Across the league, I think about half of the coaching staffs go on the bench for the National Anthem, while some wait until just before faceoff to go out there. I always liked to get out there early, eyeball the referees and see what was happening.

One time, Trotzy went long doing his between period interview with our television rightsholder Fox Sports Tennessee. His being late caused us to miss our 1:54 entry onto the bench and we had a terrible period. I think we gave up three goals that period.

"Barry, don't ever let that happen again," I told him after that awful period. "It is because you didn't make it out here for 1:54 that we gave up three goals."

It wasn't because we played badly or the other team did that well, it was because Barry was not there at the assigned time to get on the bench. Remember, I am not superstitious.

In the playoffs in 2011, they used a smoke machine as the players came out onto the ice for our home games in Nashville. There was no room in the tunnel, so the guy that was running the smoke machine was underneath the stands. I didn't see him, so each home game of the playoffs, I would throw my chewed up gum at this guy. It was dark, how was I supposed to know he was there? I didn't know that a smoke machine required an operator to be right there with it.

Finally I realized that there was a guy under there, but it was after I had already thrown about five pieces of gum at him over the course of the six home playoff games we had that year. I didn't even see him under there, but that one time I looked and saw that there was somebody moving under there. I had thrown gum in a guy's face for probably five games before I realized he was there. It was pretty funny, not to him mind you, but it was funny.

It really was dark in the building as the players came on the ice during the playoffs though, and when they added the smoke, it got dangerous. In one of our games against Vancouver, Matt Halischuk came flying out onto the ice before the game and did not see that CBC had a cameraman right there shooting video of the players. Hali skated right into the guy and smashed the camera into a million pieces. The guy ended up taking a few stitches as a result of the collision too.

Now that I have moved upstairs, I don't think that he does it anymore though. Barry is not superstitious; he would just placate my idiosyncrasies. Peter is not superstitious either. He went along with it because he was the junior member of the staff at that time, but from time to time, he would just shake his head at us and say, "You guys are nuts." He had a lot of respect, but he thought I was more nuts than anything.

Over the years, we were looking for anything to grab hold of, whether it was when we stepped on the bench or walked on the ice. Sometimes Peter and I would decide whether we were going to go down to the press room and eat. For me, it was more trying to break a routine, for Peter it was more of just him being hungry. I was more worried about keeping things going right or trying to change them up. With Peter, it was just about hunger.

Barry was always great to me, both as a boss and as a friend. A lot of assistant coaches can't say that they had a good relationship with their head coach, but

Barry is someone I will always consider a friend. He is the kind of guy who would do anything to help if he could.

He serves on the board of the Peterson for Parkinson's Foundation and is always there to help me with the golf tournaments or the pre-tournament party. And he doesn't just show up and play golf, he helps with the planning and even picks people up at the airport and brings them where they need to be. Now that I think about it, Barry really seems to like picking people up at the airport.

At the 2011 Petey's Party, Barry got up and spoke to the crowd. It was the first gathering after I stepped down from my coaching position. He said some very nice things about me and even led off with the story about me asking him to carry my bag the first time I came to interview for the position in Nashville. The story drew huge laughs from the 900 or so people in attendance that night.

Barry has been the most loyal, honest, and great friend for all of these years, and for that, I am very blessed.

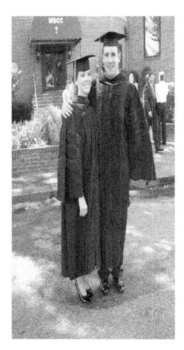

Ryan and Annie at graduation from medical school
(Peterson Family Photo)

Chapter Thirteen - Getting My Voice Back

During a game in my last season as a player, I went down to the ice in an attempt to block a shot. While I was successful in blocking that shot, I did so with my throat. It hurt – a lot. I could barely make a sound after. There was a considerable amount of swelling in the area where I was hit, and it stayed that way for a while. I continued to play after the injury occurred. It was just like I had a sore throat for a while. After all the swelling went down, the doctors checked it out, and they told me that I had a paralyzed vocal cord.

A person's vocal cords come together to make sound. One of mine was paralyzed, so the other one had to do all of the work. I had a really faint, gruff voice and nobody could hear me when I talked. I had all kinds of doctors look at me, but they all said there was nothing they could do. They just said you are going to live with it being like that. I felt like there was nothing much more I could do about it, so I just went about my life without much of a voice.

Coaching is a tough profession to be in when you can't talk very loudly, but I did the best I could with what I had. Looking back, the lack of a voice was probably a big reason I threw water bottles and rule books at referees instead of just yelling at them like most coaches do.

All those years I was coaching in Portland, I had microphones on the ice with me for practices so my players could hear me. It was really hard to communicate during games in loud buildings though.

The funny thing about my voice was if I ever yelled skate or anything, it would go high. When I coached with Team Canada as an assistant, Scott Walker who played for me in Nashville, was there. One time I tried to yell at someone, and the rest of the guys on the ice who didn't know me would ask Walks, "What's wrong with your coach?" "He sounds goofy."

One day in 2002 I was on the golf course at Legends in Franklin, TN, and I hit the ball way right. I yelled, "Fore," but nothing came out. Things were a little backed up on the course that day, and this little man came up from the group behind mine and said, "You have a paralyzed vocal cord, don't you?"

"Yes," I said.

"Well, I can fix that," he said.

That man's name was Dr. Ed Stone. He was the director of the Vanderbilt Voice Clinic in Nashville. He handled the voices of some of the biggest country music stars. Dr. Stone brought me into his office and put one of those cameras down my throat.

He said, "Sure enough, you have a paralyzed vocal cord."

My sarcastic reflex kicked in when I responded, "Thanks Doc, I already knew that."

Dr. Stone was close to retiring, so he had Dr. Mark Courey do my surgery.

During the surgery, the doctors split my throat from ear to ear. They put a hole in my voice box and put a shim in there to hold the paralyzed vocal cord closer to the other one. During the surgery, Channel 2, ABC's affiliate in Nashville, was there recording video. It must not have looked good because the cameraman fainted during the surgery while he was shooting the video. It is not a reassuring feeling when you are the patient and someone in the operating room takes a dive. On the bright side, at least it wasn't one of the medical professionals in the room. That would have been a really bad sign for me.

I was awake through the entire surgery. It was just like I was in the dentist chair, except for the small fact that no dentist I have ever been to has split my throat from ear to ear. I had to talk and make noises for them. I could feel the vibration just like a dentist drills on my teeth.

At one point, Dr. Courey told me to sing "Happy Birthday," so I sang "Happy Birthday." My voice was really high. I sounded like Mickey Mouse. The guys would have never let me live that one down.

"We don't want it there," he said, so he moved it into another position. Again, he said, sing "Happy Birthday," so I sang it again. That one was too low.

I sounded like Lou Rawls. Now that I think about it, we probably should have left it there so that I could have had a signing career to fall back on later in life.

Dr. Courey finally got the vocal cord in the right place where I sounded a lot more like Brent Peterson as opposed to Mickey Mouse or Lou Rawls. He then sewed me up and we were done.

I wasn't allowed to talk for a month after the surgery to let it heal properly.

My kids had grown up with me talking in not much more than a whisper. I had a really loud voice before I got hurt. After the month of healing had passed, one day I came downstairs and yelled, "What's going on?" They all jumped. It shocked them, and they all turned around. They had never heard me with a voice like that.

One day after that, Trotzy said we had to call the team, so we split up the names. Marty Erat was on my list, so I called Marty who was at home in the Czech Republic.

"Marty, it's Brent Peterson," I said.

He was used to my other voice, so he said, "Yeah right Vokey."

He thought it was Tomas Vokoun prank calling him, so he hung up on me.

I called him back, and he said, "Vokey, leave me alone."

Instead of letting this go on for the rest of the afternoon, I went over and told Trotzy what was going on with Marty not thinking it was really me who was the one calling him. Trotzy called Marty and told him that it was really me calling him and not Vokey playing a joke on him.

I am not sure how Marty thought that my new voice sounded anything like Tomas Vokoun though. Poor Vokey, he is so misunderstood. One day he called one of the sports talk radio stations in Nashville unannounced. Apparently they were talking about him and he wanted to chime in on the conversation. He called in on the listener line and not the station's hotline, so the call screener was a little skeptical. During that call, the screener told him that he needed to work on his Tomas Vokoun impression… and hung up on him.

It really was a miracle surgery for me. From 1989 to 2002, I could barely talk, I couldn't yell, and nobody could hear me. The sequence of events that took place for this whole process to occur is amazing. What is really unbelievable is that Dr. Stone just happened to be behind me on the very rare occasion that I hit a bad golf shot and had to attempt to yell, "Fore."

Chapter Fourteen - Golf, My Other Favorite Sport

It seems as though a great deal of my life has been hitting inanimate objects with a crooked stick. I have made my living as a hockey player and coach, and ever since I was a teenager, I have loved the sport of golf.

I started playing golf back in the 1970s when I was about 16. I got a job at a golf course cutting greens and doing all of that kind of work. After a while, my boss came up to me and told me that he needed a night waterman. There were no automatic sprinklers back then, so you had to move the sprinklers around the course to make sure everything was watered. I did that during the summers when I was playing junior hockey. I would sleep all day and be the waterman at the golf course at night.

This was a private country club, and one of the benefits of working there was that they let the employees golf on Mondays. When I started, I was never very good, but I really enjoyed playing. When the kids were born, I did not have a lot of time to play, but as they got older, I got back to playing more and more.

PGA touring professional Peter Jacobsen has been a great friend of mine for over 30 years. Peter's wife grew up across the street from Tami in Portland. Peter turned pro in 1974, and I turned pro in 1978. He would always be at his in-laws, and I would always be at my in-laws, so that is how we got to know each other.

One day he was playing in the Oregon Open. He was already a touring pro at this point, but he always came back to Portland for the Oregon Open, and he said, "Come walk with me tomorrow." I didn't even know him very well at that point. That day, he was a little bit under the weather and didn't have a caddy. After the first hole, I said, "Peter give me your bag." I carried his bag and caddied for him the rest of the way. He thought I was a great guy and we have been really close friends ever since.

Every year, Peter held his Fred Meyer Challenge in Portland. It was a big tournament. A few days before the tournament, I would go with him to Denver to the International Tournament at Castle Pines. We would get all of the guys that got beaten on Friday and Saturday. The International used the Modified Stableford scoring system, so if the players got beaten and did not make the final round, they would usually always come over to Portland and play in Peter's tournament.

My job was to get with the players and arrange things for them, get their airfare or whatever they needed on short notice so that they would come to Portland to play in the Pro-Am on Sunday.

Every year, Peter would have his friends host a player. We would pick them up at the airport and we would take care of them for the four days. I had Curtis Strange for four years, Ben Crenshaw, Steve Elkington, and Scott McCarron as well. They were all great guys.

One year, I took care of Tom Kite and did not talk to him for a year afterwards, but the next year when he saw me at the International, he came up to me and said, "Hey Brent, how are you doing?" He remembered me. That's amazing.

I was still playing in the NHL during the first few years of the tournament and a lot of the golfers knew me, so whenever they saw me, they would say, "He shoots, he scores." Apparently they did not know a lot about hockey, because if they did, they would know that I did not shoot and score very much. They would tease me about being a hockey player. Jay Haas still remembers me, and when he sees me, he says something about hockey.

While I was coaching the Winter Hawks, Peter became the pro to help design the Oregon Golf Club, a beautiful and challenging course perched on a hill overlooking the Willamette Valley. One day, he invited me to the club for a game of golf. We entered the mahogany locker room where he showed me to his own locker. Right next to his was another locker with my name on it. I said, "Peter, you can't do that," to which he replied, "I can't? Oh, yes I can." I enjoyed those years of membership at that club, as did my family.

Being such a jokester, Peter said to Tami, "I just love your husband. If he was a girl, I would marry him." She reminded him that I was already taken.

I love the challenge of golf. I have been known to play 36 holes in a day by noon. I just like it. I could play all day, every day. I don't play Sundays because of church and family time. The other six days I try to get out as much as I can. Now I play as much golf as I can because I'm not sure that I am going to be able to play as much as I go along. Sometimes when I was locked up, I couldn't even swing a club.

We don't get too many off days in the winter, so I never really played much in the winter. I probably average only once per month in the winter. From the time we got beaten out of the playoffs until September, I probably played five times a week.

When we were on road trips, Pete Rogers, the Predators' equipment manager, and I played if we could. Rain, sleet, snow, it didn't matter; we got out there if we had an opportunity.

I have great friends who I play with, and we go on golf trips together. The past 10 years we have gone on some great trips and had a lot of fun. Tami has been great to let me go to those places. Unfortunately, as the symptoms of Parkinson's progressed, it did not look like I was going to be able to go on many more golf trips.

Over the years, I have been fortunate enough to play on some of the best courses in North America, a lot of the ones the PGA Tour plays each year. I have played Pebble Beach, Pinehurst, Whisper Rock, Riviera, Doral, Winged Foot, Medina, Kapalua, and Sawgrass just to name a few.

Pebble is probably the most scenic. Pinehurst is beautiful. In my opinion, Number Two is not the best one of the courses there. I think Number Four is probably the best, but they play the U.S. Open on Number Two.

The 17th hole at the TPC Sawgrass is the famed island hole that always makes the Players Championship tournament so interesting each and every year. The 17th is pretty cool. You have to hit a good shot to get it on the green. I hit it short and missed the green once, putting it in the water. I don't feel too badly about it though. A lot of the pros do it every year too. The other two times I played that hole, I put the ball on the green though, so two out of three isn't too bad I don't think.

I have a bucket list of places that I still want to play. I haven't played Augusta, Cypress Point, Pine Valley, or Whistling Straits. Those would probably be at the top of the list of courses I would jump at the chance of playing them if the opportunities present themselves.

The NHL's lockout of 2004-05 gave me an excuse to play a lot more golf than normal. That was when I played the best golf of my life. I am an 11 handicap now, but I got down to a two during the lockout.

The lockout was when I recorded both of my career holes-in-one.

My first hole-in-one came in the morning group on hole number 16 at the Vanderbilt Legends Club in Franklin, Tennessee, just south of Nashville. I hit an eight iron from 150 yards, and it went right in, much to my delight.

The second hole-in-one also came at Legends. That one was on hole number five. I hit a five iron from 180 yards.

It was a really slow day, and since I like to play fast, I was a little bit irritated. There was a group on the green, our group was on the tee, and there was a group coming up behind us. Since I was frustrated at how slow the group in front of us was playing, I hit my shot as they were walking off of the green.

Thinking back, I am lucky that I did not hit that one too long, or else there is a chance that I would have hit one of them with the ball.

When I hit the shot, one of the guys in my group said, "That one is going to be close Petey." When it landed and went in, we all went crazy. The guys walking off the green saw it, my group, of course, saw it, and the foursome behind us saw it too, so there were a lot of witnesses to that one.

The two holes-in-one came within three months of each other and I haven't been close since.

The timing of the holes-in-one was interesting. I had been diagnosed with Parkinson's a year earlier and had just gone public with my diagnosis. After such a difficult year, having positive things like the holes-in-one happen really gave me a positive outlook on things at a time when I was still coming out of feeling very sorry for myself for a long time.

Chapter Fifteen - Coaching Brad

Most people think that my last head coaching job was in Portland prior to heading for Nashville, but the lockout of the NHL's 2004-05 season provided a special opportunity for me to run my own bench for what turned out to be the last time.

For one season, I was the head coach of the club hockey team at Middle Tennessee State University. What made that gig really special was the fact that my son Brad was one of the players on that team.

John Latreille was in charge of coaching the MTSU club team, and during the lockout, they all came to me and asked if I would like to help out with the team. John had coached Brad at Centennial High School for two seasons after we moved to Nashville from Portland. He was a Canadian guy who came down here to work at the Saturn automotive plant. He retired from Saturn and had his own handyman business doing home improvements.

Since I had a lot of time, and I didn't have much scouting to do, I decided I would go and take the team over and John would help me. He was a great guy and we had a great year the one season we coached together. We went 33-1.

John passed away late in 2012 after a long and courageous battle with brain cancer. He was a great friend and he made a big impact on hockey in the Middle Tennessee area.

Club hockey is not like the major college hockey played at schools like Boston College or Michigan State. There is no recruiting, no facilities, or big budgets given from the schools. It is pretty much just kids who go to that school and can play a little hockey get together and form a team.

We didn't have any money. We just scraped it together. MTSU gave us a little money, but guys had to pay their own way on the club team. There was no rink on the campus in Murfreesboro, so the guys had to drive 45 minutes each way to the rink in Franklin for practices and home games.

There were a bunch of characters on that team. One guy would always stay down on the ice for way too long after he took a hit. One game it happened again right before the end of a period. When we went into the locker room at the intermission the guys were all sitting there, so I decided to have a little fun with him. So in front of the team, I said. "Hey, my wife is up in the stands and she is pretty good looking, if I get her down on the ice to perform CPR on you, would that make you get up any faster?"

The guys on the team were just dying laughing at that. It is always good to try and keep the guys loose with some humor, but it is even better when you can use it to deliver a message as well.

I got all the guys to buy in that season. We went up to Michigan and beat several of the teams that had won the national championships on the club level.

Unfortunately, despite our great record, we were not voted to play in the nationals that season though.

We were disappointed that we were not voted in the top three of our conference. Only the top three teams from each conference were voted into the nationals. We were voted fourth in our conference. We had already beaten the three teams that went ahead of us from our conference. It didn't go by the record. It went by the voting.

I called the head guy and he said, "Who are you?"

I said, "It doesn't matter who I am, but there was a travesty going on here. It's not fair."

He said, "Too bad."

I explained it to him, but it turned out to be a waste of time. The poor kids worked so hard, and that was the only year they were going to have my time and me. Some of them were seniors, and they weren't going to get a chance to play for a national championship. They went to Florida, Texas, Michigan and we beat them all, but the other teams got in by the votes. The coaches voted, and because we had never done anything before, when it came time to vote, some of them didn't realize that we had a good team that year. We didn't play all of the other teams, but that year, we beat the number two, three, and five teams; we were fourth. We never got to see the first place team, and they didn't even win the national championship.

Getting the opportunity to coach Brad was cool. During my years as a player and a coach, it was impossible for me to coach or work with any of the kids' sports teams when they were younger, so for this opportunity to come along when it did was one of the very few good things about the NHL being shut down for an entire season.

Brad is a great kid and was a really talented player. Physically, he matured late. He was 21 before he was where he should have been at 17. He is a talented guy and could go out now and skate with the Predators players and hold his own any day. He couldn't play in the NHL, but he could go out in a practice and be just as good as a lot of the guys. He couldn't play in the games because he is smallish, but he absolutely has great skills. He loves the game and loves being around the game.

But, I couldn't let the other players on the team think I was favoring my own son, even though Brad was by far the best player. He was a talented player, but sometimes he didn't always play hockey the way I liked it to be played, like in terms of teamwork for example. I was hard on him, but he still loves me.

One game, there was a too many men on the ice penalty and the referee came over to the bench. Brad wasn't on the ice when the penalty was called. I said, "16 is serving it." The referee said it had to be someone on the ice. I said, "It doesn't matter, 16 is serving it."

The referee and I had a little set-to, and finally I got him to agree to let 16 go serve it. In case you were wondering, Brad wore number 16. He wasn't on the ice and had nothing to do with it, I was just mad at him. But when I made him go over and serve that penalty, boy was he ever mad at me.

He got over it though. Soon after the penalty expired, he got the puck and went coast-to-coast and scored a goal. When he came back to the bench, he just glared at me.

Now Brad works as one of the equipment guys with the Predators. Having the chance to be around him at the rink every day is great. Again, I missed a lot of games, school activities, and the like when he was younger, but having this time together as adults is something not a lot of people get to experience with their children.

I make him continue to go to school. I told him I will pay for it, but you have to go and finish your school. He takes one or two classes at a time because he is so busy. Some days, he picks up the team at the airport at 3:00 in the morning and then he has to be at school at 8:00. He is still plugging away. He has to get that degree. He might never use it, but he has to get that degree. It could be the matter of a door open or a door shut. Once you have that degree, it is yours forever. I joke with him that he is on the 12-year program, but he is on his way to getting there, and I am very proud of him for doing it.

Chapter Sixteen - Meet the Petersons

It was a freezing January night in Hartford. Tami's mother, Marla, had just arrived to stay with her in case our third child decided to enter this world a little early while I was on a road trip. I had just fallen into a deep sleep only to be awakened by Marla, who informed me that Tami was in labor. I responded by rolling over and going back to sleep. After going through this twice before, I thought it had to be a false alarm. She convinced me that it was the real thing, so we bundled up the boys and took them to a friend's house. The trip to the hospital was over frozen and snow-covered streets. In the back seat, my mother-in-law, in rather strong terms, suggested that it wasn't necessary to wait for signal lights to turn green given the fact that it was snowing and that there was not another living creature in sight.

After much effort on Tami's part, our darling baby girl Kristin made her arrival into this world. This was before ultrasound testing, so I was excited to have a daughter. I still feel the same way every time I see her. She and I have had a very special bond and she still has me firmly wrapped around all of her fingers.

We sent her off to college in Utah. Several years later, the time came when she decided to bring her "boyfriend" home to meet the parents. I don't know who was more nervous, Aaron or me. He had told Kristin that he was very concerned about meeting me in particular.

His visit closely resembled that of the *Meet the Parents* series of movies featuring Ben Stiller and Robert De Niro.

Kristin and Aaron had arrived in Nashville a day before I returned from Detroit. At the time, we had been having some trouble with the guest bathroom toilet. Instead of fixing it, Tami just turned off the water and forgot to turn it on again before the kids got home. Aaron was in the bathroom a very long time and finally came out asking for a bucket. He said he needed it to flush the toilet. It was just a little embarrassing for them all.

I arrived back home late afternoon the next day, and after introductions, I asked Aaron if he knew how to use a barbeque, as Tami was preparing dinner and steaks were on the menu. Aaron assured me that he knew how to use it, so I headed upstairs to unpack and do the same routine that I followed after each road trip. In the meantime, Tami had elevated the temperature of the grill to burn off some old ash. Aaron put the steaks on the grill and closed the cover. When I came back downstairs, I saw Aaron with horror on his face and showing less facial hair and eyebrows than he had when I had originally met him. The steaks had only been on for a few minutes, and when he raised the hood, a blast erupted. I said, "I thought you said you knew how to barbeque." Aaron was horrified and sat there picking off the charred parts of the steaks.

I had to go to bed a little early, as we had another game the next day. The kids stayed up, and of course, Aaron used the bathroom before he went to bed. I got up at 5:30 the next morning, came downstairs and looked up at the ceiling of our living room only to see it bowed way down and ready to break open. Brown water was dripping off of it. I yelled for Tami who came running down the stairs thinking that Tucker, our dog, had gotten sick. She went into action and called John Latreille, who had come to our rescue more than once, and told him our problem. He came immediately and decided to poke holes in the sagging ceiling before the whole thing caved in and caused an even bigger mess than we already had on our hands.

It was not a pretty sight. Brown water spewed everywhere soaking the carpet. John had moved the furniture, but not the big screen TV. The cascading torrent missed it by inches. Thank goodness I had to leave (again) and left them to start cleaning up the mess. The kids were still sleeping, and when Aaron found out what had happened, he was stunned. Tami reassured him it wasn't his fault that the toilet just kept running after he had used it and didn't shut off, resulting in a flood of water that ran under the baseboards to the floor below.

It was then that Aaron decided that he thought it was time for him to go back to Utah. After that, everything that went wrong, like if the garage door stopped working or a rock hit the car's windshield, we blamed it on Aaron. He took the ribbing well. He had no choice, and it didn't end there.

I went to the rink and told all of the guys about what had happened. They were ruthless when they met Aaron for the first time. "So you're the guy who wrecked Peterson's house, eh?" came from everyone in the locker room when I took him down there. Mitch Korn showed Aaron all of the expensive electronic equipment that operates everything and quickly said to him, "Don't touch anything."

Aaron later went to visit Tami at the beauty salon where she worked and he was told he was not allowed to use the bathroom.

Well, Aaron survived his initiation to our family and eventually became our son-in-law. I figured he deserved as tough a time as I had received from Tami's dad when I asked him if I could marry his daughter. Being a banker, he gave me the third degree. Fortunately for me though, I never broke anything.

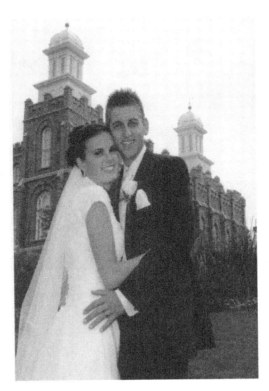

Kristin and Aaron at their wedding (Peterson Family Photo)

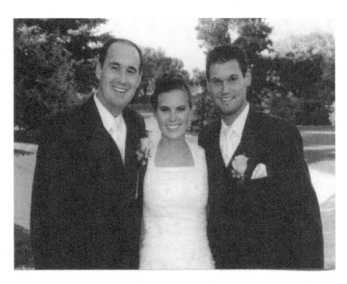

Ryan, Kristin, and Brad at Kristin's Wedding (Peterson Family Photo)

Chapter Seventeen - My Last Year Behind the Bench

Very early on in the 2010-11 season, probably October or November, it became apparent that my time as a coach was close to being over. I knew that the end was coming at some point, but it was still an extremely difficult thing to accept when the end actually became a reality.

Every year since the Parkinson's diagnosis, I had been fine and just went along doing my job, but just that last year, I had no balance. I was rigid more often too. Making things worse was the fact that I wasn't sleeping well either. The doctors tried different medications and they worked at times, but other times they did not do well enough to make much of a difference. I just couldn't do the job of an associate coach for an NHL team. I couldn't keep up with the pace. I really tried my best to keep up, but it just was not happening.

Being tired all the time was not just draining me physically; the mental toll it took on me was just as bad, if not worse.

When I was on the ice with the team during practice I fell a couple of times. I had hoped that no one noticed. No one said anything, so I am not sure if they didn't notice or were just trying to look the other way. Whether or not the others saw me, I knew that things were not going in the right direction with regard to my health.

I was getting in the way of the players on the ice. It was dangerous for both me and for the players. When I was fine, I was fine, but more times than not, I was not fine. It was very random times when I would get locked up. When I locked up, I couldn't even move.

Things got really scary one day in practice.

We played in Detroit October 30th. We were short a defenseman, so we dressed Wade Belak as our sixth defenseman that night. Wade was a defenseman early in his career but was moved to forward. He did not play much for us that season, but he was a great guy to have around the locker room even though he rarely got in for us that season.

I was in charge of the defense, and I did not play Wade at all in the game in Detroit. I know it was hard on him, but he took it like a pro.

A few days later in practice, I couldn't get out of his way and we collided. I was lying on the ice and Wade skated over to me and said, "That's what you get for not playing me, don't ever do that again."

He was just kidding of course, and it was funny for everyone, but the experience was a real eye-opener.

In November, I went to Trotzy and said, "Barry, I don't know how much longer I can do this. I am locked up more often. I don't sleep. I am tired all the time."

I couldn't do all the on the ice stuff. I could still do all the other stuff like watching film and developing game plans, but that was not enough. Assistant coaches have to work with the guys on the ice before and after practice. Not being able to do those kinds of things was not fair to the team.

Late in November we had a home game against the New York Rangers. I was sick that day and just couldn't make it to the game, so that was the first game I ever missed as a coach. I missed another one as well, so after not missing any games in 20 years of coaching, I missed two in 2010-11.

During the games I missed, Peter took the responsibility of changing the defense. When I returned from my illness, I told Barry that it might be a good idea if we leave the "D" with Peter. He knew that I was struggling, so he said that was fine.

I didn't want to hurt the team. I could have kept going and probably done a pretty good job with the defense, but I wanted to make sure we were going on all cylinders. We had a good team. I thought we could have had a good chance and I didn't want to be the guy to mess it up. I continued to handle the penalty killing units.

Every year around January or so, David would talk with the coaches about a contract for the next season. He always started at the top with Trotzy.

David went to Barry and asked if he wanted his assistants back, and he said yes.

David then came in and offered me a contract for the next season. I thought I was very honest and forward with him. I could have taken the contract and made good money by making my way through coaching as best as I could.

I said, "David, I am not 100%. I can't do the job you are asking me to do. So this is what has to happen; I am probably going off the ice in a month or two and try to make it as long as I can."

I didn't want to take money that I wasn't going to earn. Not long after that, my doctor told me it was time to get off of the ice for good. That was in March, and we still had a little over a month left in the regular season plus the playoffs. I tried to stay on the ice as long as I could so there would be some continuity, but in March, my time had come.

People started asking me why I was not on the ice at practice and the morning skates, but we wanted the focus to be on the team and not me, so when asked, I just said that was doing more work with video and stuff.

We finished the regular season in fifth place in the Western Conference and faced the Anaheim Ducks in the first round of the playoffs. That was the sixth time in seven seasons that we had made the playoffs. Unfortunately for us, we had not won a playoff series in our first five trips to the postseason.

For us, the sixth time was the charm though, as we were able to beat Anaheim in six games.

For me, the thrill of the playoffs was amazing. Playoffs are when you are really excited. Once we made the playoffs and were doing well in the playoffs, I was fine health-wise. I knew that was going to be my last kick at the can. The guys played well and we pulled out the series win.

David Legwand scored an empty-net goal in Game 6 to clinch both the game and the first playoff series win in franchise history. Game 6 was at home in Bridgestone Arena in Nashville, so when Leggy scored that goal, all of the fans that had been with us from the start through some lean years finally had something to celebrate. It was so loud in there during the games, but when Leggy scored and we knew we were going to win, I thought the roof was going to blow off of the arena. That was awesome.

We played the Vancouver Canucks in the second round, but unfortunately, we lost to them in six games.

After that series ended, Tami told me that I looked like a truck had run over me. We had made two trips to Anaheim and also made two to Vancouver, so in addition to the pressure of the playoffs, we spent a lot of time on planes flying around North America.

A couple of days after we were eliminated by Vancouver, we had our break up day where the players and coaches meet with the media to wrap the season. During David's press conference, he announced that I would not be back as a member of the coaching staff for the next season. It was not a big surprise to anyone who was in attendance that day, but it was still a tough thing for David to do.

David and I always had a good relationship, and making things worse for him was the fact that his late father Bud also had Parkinson's, so it was doubly difficult for him to get through the announcement. He is always so steady in everything he does; to see him get choked up like he did was really touching.

After he made the announcement, he called me up to the dais, and the media gave me a nice round of applause, which was very kind of them. The media contingency in Nashville is not all that big, so I knew just about everyone in there that day.

A few weeks after that press conference, David, Barry, and I met and came up with a new title of hockey operations advisor. My mind still works, but some days I just can't get around. When I feel good, I will go on the road with the team. If I am not feeling my best, I will hang back and find other things to do. Luckily David and Barry have been great to work with and great to my family, so I am so thankful that they were willing to create this position to accommodate me and keep me around.

Chapter Eighteen - The DBS Decision

For a few years, I kicked around the idea of undergoing the procedure called Deep Brain Stimulation in hopes of alleviating some of the symptoms as my Parkinson's progressed.

A few people suggested to me that I would have a better quality of life and I would not have to take as many medications, as there were many side effects associated with them. It is a lot to go through to get to that, but many people had called me and talked about how it had worked for them, as did former Major League Baseball player Ben Petrick.

Ben was diagnosed with Parkinson's at 22-years-old, and the amazing thing is that he managed to play a couple of years of Major League Baseball with Parkinson's. After leaving baseball, Ben underwent DBS. The results were impressive. He came to my foundation's dinner in 2011 and showed a video of the before and after of what the procedure did for him.

Ben underwent DBS only to suffer an infection, which required the electrode sensors to be removed. But he knew what the DBS could do for him because he had felt the results during the surgery.

DBS is a very involved process and it is not without risks. I don't remember ever saying that I would never consider the option, but Tami claims that I had and we know she is always right.

Initially there were two reasons why I didn't want the operation. First, I wasn't ready for another surgery, especially one as elaborate as DBS. Only a few years before, prior to our son Ryan's graduation from medical school in Memphis, I experienced a sudden stabbing pain in my kidney area only to learn that there was a walnut sized stone lodged in my kidney.

A treatment to break up the stone was attempted, but that didn't make even a scratch on it, so the doctor decided that they would have to go in surgically. An interventional radiologist, who performed the technique, determined exactly where the stone was located. They opened the kidney and could see this massive chunk of mineral. Once again they attempted to break it up with their device. Once again, it failed. So they took a drill to it, broke it up, and removed it.

There were no sutures. We were told that once the drain was removed, the tissue would heal on its own.

Home we went, and we followed all of the medical instructions. We were anxious to get through this with family coming from Oregon and Canada for the graduation. When the drain tube was removed, we did not expect what was to happen next. I began to urinate out of the hole in my back.

I had no control over it. It just kept coming. Tami took heavy towels and wrapped them tightly around me. She called the surgeon who said we would probably have to go back into surgery. Just what I needed, right? When she checked me again after loosening the tight binding, we were astonished to see that the flow had stopped.

My buddies came to check up on me and laughingly said it was too bad there wasn't snow on the ground outside so that I could go out and write my name in it with my back. They had a good laugh at my expense. We did make the graduation on time.

The second reason I didn't want DBS was because I didn't think that I was so far along with my condition that I needed to seek such a drastic treatment.

Just in the last eight months before the procedure, my condition declined quite noticeably. I had a lot of rigidity a lot longer during the day and more times during the night. I think I would have been in good shape if the disease had not progressed to the point it had, but it had gotten worse, and it was not going to get any better on its own.

I would sleep off and on – an hour here and an hour there, and maybe catch a catnap in the afternoon. I don't know if it was the disease or the medications, probably a little bit of both. I just couldn't sleep. I got to bed at 10:00 or 11:00 and I'd wake up and it would be 12:15. I would wander the halls and try not to wake everyone up. Tami can sleep through a tornado. I would come down and read or watch TV and I would fall asleep on the couch at 3:00 or 4:00 a.m.

Just a couple of weeks before I underwent Deep Brain Stimulation, I was wandering around the house and ended up in the kitchen looking for something to eat. I always had a good appetite, and the Parkinson's did not change that. While rooting around the pantry, I found three large Hershey's chocolate bars.

Since there were three of them, I didn't think that anyone would notice if one of them was not there. So, each night for the next few days, I would wake up and then find myself in the kitchen and eating some of the chocolate. After a few days, I finally made my way through them all.

At about 8:00 the night before Thanksgiving, I was sitting in the living room watching the Predators play a game in Minnesota, when all of a sudden Tami yells from the kitchen, "Brent, did you eat these chocolate bars?"

As it turns out, she needed those to make some pies for Thanksgiving and was not pleased at all to find out that I was responsible for them disappearing.

Oh well, the stores were still open and she was able to replace them.

Even though everything was tough on me, I could almost learn to deal with all of it except for the constant state of fatigue. All of the physical problems are tough to deal with, but not being able to sleep not only affects you physically, but the mental challenge of being exhausted all the time was just too much to deal with on an everyday basis.

More times than not, shaving was an adventure. I had started using an electric razor more or else I would have needed sutures every morning.

Something had to be done. I was not getting better, and things were progressing for the worse rather quickly. I still felt like I had a lot of good years ahead of me.

Not everyone with Parkinson's is a candidate for DBS. There is a lot of testing that needs to be done in order to make sure that a good result is likely for a Parkinson's patient.

The tough part was that I had to go off my meds totally for the first day of the tests. That was a tough two-day stretch. They tested my walking and they tested my brainpower. They basically test your IQ. It is a three-hour test. You have to walk up and down and jump, and all of that is without your medications. Then you have to come back the next day and they do all of the tests over again with your meds. They want to see if the medications help. The only way the DBS will help is if the medications help you. You need more and more medications as time passes, and they eventually lose their effectiveness. Another downside is that they have so many side effects.

I did really well with the physical tests that they put me through. The doctors said that being a former professional athlete, and the fact that I was still in reasonably good shape physically were good signs that I would be able to withstand the physical toll that DBS would take on me.

Then came the mental evaluations. The IQ tests were tough. They tested my memory.

First they showed me pictures of 20 people, and then a minute later, they had to test the short-term memory by asking me to tell them which ones were in the first 10. I finally said, "Lady, I don't really care."

She flipped them over and I went, "No, no, no, yes, yes, yes..."

I said, "Lady I don't really care if I pass this or not, so get on with it."

After that test, they moved on to another one where I had to name as many animals as I could in a minute. You should have heard of some of the ones I came up with.

"Lion, tiger, giraffe, anteater…." That was all I had.

I was so tired and so tired of being there, I just couldn't come up with anything else.

The best part about it was when the doctor called me. He said, "You passed all of your tests, but you didn't do very well on your animals."

The next time I was in his office, Dr. Davis asked me to name some more animals.

"Lion, tiger, cow, giraffe…"

Again, I couldn't think of any more animals. He basically said that there is something wrong with me because I couldn't name more than five animals. It was then that Tami chimed in with, "Brent, didn't your mother ever take you to the zoo?"

Then he told me to name as many words that begin with the letter A within a minute.

"Ant, asshole…"

Seriously, that was all I could think of at that point.

He said, "Can't we do any better than that?"

I said I couldn't think of anything else. I didn't pass my animal or my words that begin with A tests.

Finally, he said, "We will still let you be a candidate for DBS even though you are a dummy."

So this dummy went through the four-stage process of DBS in December of 2011.

Chapter Nineteen - Undergoing DBS

Let me make one thing clear – DBS is not a cure for Parkinson's. A lot of people think that it is a cure, but unfortunately it is not. I still have Parkinson's and I will always have Parkinson's, but the DBS has made a world of difference in dealing with my symptoms.

I think the surgery is misunderstood. Everybody thinks it is a cure for Parkinson's, but it has nothing to do with that. All it does is get you off of your medications. The medications do the same things as the DBS, but the medications don't last forever, you need more and more each year. I almost thought I could cure myself by having this thing. I am down from about 20 pills a day to five at the most. Before DBS, I couldn't sleep well at night. 50% of Parkinson's patients have numerous side effects, depression, and all kinds of other things. This system blocks the bad signals the Parkinson's gives you. So now I only have to take a little dopamine. If I don't take it, I still get locked up like I did before.

At first I didn't think that I was that bad, but looking back, it has been a long trek and I had been getting progressively worse at a pretty fast rate.

At Vanderbilt University Medical Center, they do DBS in a four-step process; three surgeries and the last part is where it is turned on and begins to function.

In the first surgery, they shaved my head, drilled four screws into my head, and finally, they marked my brain. Those screws are used to hold the halo in place when they do the second step of the procedure.

As involved as drilling four screws into one's head sounds, it was just an outpatient procedure, and I was home that day. The whole process took somewhere between 90 minutes and two hours. The best part was that even though I just had four screws drilled into the top of my head, I didn't really have anything in the way of pain or discomfort.

The next week was the second stage of DBS and that was a tough one. I had to go off my meds at 6:00 the night before. For this one, I had to be awake. They gave me six or seven shots to the top of my skull to numb it up, and then they drilled two more holes in the top of my head. Then they put the halo on. It has four holes and has something attaching it in the middle. It has two holes on the top where the electrodes go into the brain.

In the second procedure, I could feel them drilling into my head. I had to be awake, so all I had was a bunch of little needles giving me the local anesthesia on my head. They were drilling on my head, and I could feel it when they went through. It was pretty weird. The best way I can describe it is that it felt similar to when a dentist is drilling on my teeth. You know they are there and what they are doing, but the anesthesia prevents you from feeling any pain. It was like drilling into a board and feeling when you go through. It didn't hurt, but you could feel what they were doing.

Thankfully, my hair has grown back where they drilled the holes, but I can still feel the bumps in the spots where the screws were located.

After, they hooked it up to a computer. I was awake so they could have me move my hands, throw the ball, and other physical things.

The people in the operating room were throwing the ball with me, and meanwhile the doctor was putting electrodes down into my brain! It was pretty wild. They also put the wires behind my ear in a big heap because they had not put the thing in my chest yet. They had it turned on to make sure it was working and that I was moving correctly.

At one point, I said, "Do you guys want to hear a joke?" Everybody in the operating room stopped and I told a joke. Everybody laughed, and then they all went back to work.

I could move my head a little bit because it wasn't confined completely, but they made sure I stayed a little still. Everybody said what if you go flailing away, but I couldn't. You are right on the edge. You are awake, but you are right on the edge of going out. They have to get you loosened up to be able to talk with them.

The second procedure lasted about five hours and I had to stay overnight. I wasn't feeling too great that night.

The only person they let in the night of the second surgery was Trotzy. It was a Tuesday night and the Predators had played a home game that night. He came by Vanderbilt to see me after the game. I was hurting, but Barry came in to visit me. That really meant a lot to have him there.

I thought I would never go home the next day, but when I woke up the next morning, I felt pretty good and went home.

I couldn't really do much of anything for a week after that procedure. You have to be really careful. If you get any kind of infection anywhere, they have to pull everything out. You can't get any water in there, so I couldn't shower. I had to watch what I did with my head too, and that was easier said than done because my balance was, and still is, not all that great.

The next week, they cut the hole in my chest and put the battery pack into my chest. They pulled the wires behind my ear and down my neck and hooked them up to the battery pack. I was not awake at all for the third one.

My head hurt more than anything because they had to pull the skin away from my head and put the wires through, around the back of my ear and down my neck to be able to attach it to the battery pack.

You wake up from the head down, so when I came out of the surgery, all I could think of was I had to pee. Tami and Kristin were the only ones in there, so they scrambled to try and find something for me to pee into so that there wasn't a giant mess in the bed.

Poor Kristin, through all of this, she saw a whole lot more of me that day than she probably ever expected to.

The day that was really tough was the day of the fourth procedure when I had to go in with no meds. I could not get dressed that morning. Tami and Kristin had to put my shoes and socks on for me. That was the day that they turned it on. I could not take my meds after 6:00 the night before. When I got up in the morning I could not move.

We could not have done this without Kristin and her husband Aaron. They had stayed in Utah after graduating from Utah State University, but they decided to move back to Nashville for a year to help with things as my condition worsened.

They were great during the whole month-long DBS process. With all of the media following the procedure, at times Kristin stepped up and told the reporters and cameras the updates. It was such a blessing to have her there so that Tami could focus on me and Kristin could take care of anything else that needed to be done. It is great that my daughter has my back like that.

A month or so before the DBS process started, Tami and Kristin were handing out the candy to the trick-or-treaters on Halloween. Kristin was wearing one of my old hockey jerseys that night. One kid who was about eight or nine came up to the door and saw Kristin wearing a hockey jersey with the number 12 on it.

The kid said to his mother, "Hey mom, that girl is wearing Mike Fisher's jersey."

In a nice tone, Kristin replied back, "No it isn't, that's Brent Peterson's jersey."

Then the mom went on to let him know that someone other than Mike Fisher had worn the number 12 in the NHL before.

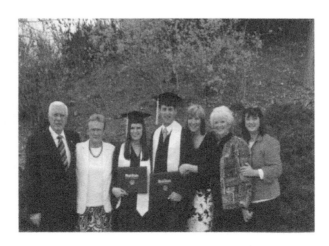

Kristin and Aaron following their graduation from
Utah State University (Peterson Family Photo)

Chapter Twenty - Post DBS

I would do DBS all over again because it was worth it, but at times when I was going through it, I would sometimes say to myself, "Why am I doing this?" It was a tough process.

It has given me everything back.

I am not exaggerating when I say this, but DBS really saved my life by giving me my life back. Prior to the procedure I was going downhill quickly, and now I still have Parkinson's, but Parkinson's no longer has me.

It is a night and day difference. I am pretty lucky I was able to do it and do it when I was still young. I didn't want to do it until about a year before it was performed. At that time, I finally realized I wasn't getting better, and my wife said, "Hey if you don't do it now, you are going to miss all these years where you could be doing so many things."

There were so many things that could go wrong, and things do go wrong - they just don't really tell you about them. The reason they don't tell you about them is that if they did, no one would do the surgeries!

They tell you the serious things that could go wrong. They tell you that there is a one percent chance you could have an aneurysm and die right there on the table. That I could handle – if I died right there on the table, I wouldn't know the difference.

They don't tell you that there is a 100% chance you are going to have a headache from where they pull the skin away from your skull to get the wires through there and it is going to hurt like hell for about four months. I can't turn my neck because I have the wires there. I can still feel the wire behind my ear. I guess since I can still feel it lying right behind my ear, I will be able to feel it for the rest of my life.

There were four camera crews with reporters following me every step of the way through the DBS procedures. At times it was tough having them around, but as a family we made the decision that it was the right thing to do in order to document everything in hopes of raising awareness about Parkinson's and to give some hope to the people that are going through this as well.

After we got to the third week, Tami said she didn't want to do it with all of the cameras following us anymore. I told her that we had gone this far and we needed to see this through to the finish in order to raise awareness. They were interviewing us constantly, and it wasn't just one interview each time. We had to sit and talk and tell the same stories to all four crews. It was tiring and time consuming, but I knew that we were doing the right thing by having so many people following us.

It raised a lot of awareness. I know it was tough on Tami and the rest of the family. You are doing brain surgery. You are going to have some problems. When it was turned on and it started working, it made all of the sacrifices worth it.

We went in for the fourth procedure where they turn the unit on and got all of the camera crews there when they turned it on. What everyone saw on TV was not what really happened though. The doctors turned it on and they put me out in front of the cameras. I hammed it up a little for them. For the TSN crew I acted like John Belushi in *Animal House* shuffling my feet from side to side like I was ready to run through a wall or something.

The way I was acting was not normal for me, and the sit-down interviews right after were an adventure as well.

After they turned the device on, four people wanted to interview me separately. So, I had to do four separate interviews of five minutes each. I told one of the crews, "All I want to do is go home and go for a walk with my wife and my dog, and then I want to go for a walk with my dog and my wife."

What the cameras didn't see was when we were in the room with the family and the doctor. It was almost like two totally different things. The cameras only saw the results of the stimulation.

Right when they turned it on, I was looking at Kristin and Brad. They were looking back at me, and all of a sudden my vision went blurry three different times. When I said that I couldn't see, all Tami could think about was that we have gone through all of this and I ended up blind.

They switched it back off and Dr. Conrad came into the room. I went blind three more times. He can control all kinds of things; whether I go blind, whether I was nauseous, whether I was numb, just about anything.

He was trying to find the right place in the brain to stimulate the areas that would help me. There is a hair rod in my head that has four levels on it; A, B, C, and D. He was trying to find the place in the brain where the bad area was. When they turn it on, it makes a pulsation in that spot.

He tried the right hand first. That was my bad one, and at first it didn't work. We were worried that the whole thing wasn't going to work at all. Then he tried to make the left hand work. That one worked well, which was a relief to all of us. Mentally, I don't know how I could have handled it if nothing worked after going through a month's worth of procedures.

Then he told me to get up and try to walk. I knew it worked right away when I got up and walked, because when we went in there, I could barely shuffle my feet into the hospital. A couple of hours before, I couldn't even get myself dressed, and now I was up walking around the office.

My right hand didn't work until about two hours after we left the hospital. We were in Noshville, a local deli not far from Vanderbilt. Tami was there with my son-in-law Aaron. When Kristin saw that I was doing well, she went to work at the arena.

We were sitting there at lunch, and all of a sudden, I was like, "Oh my gosh, oh my gosh... it is working, it is working."

I felt a tingling sensation in my right arm, and all of a sudden I just got up and walked out of the door of the restaurant. Aaron and Tami didn't know what to do but try and chase me down and see where I was going and what I planned to do.

The team was in Washington for a road game against the Capitals that night. That trip was that season's dad's trip, so all of the players' fathers were on the trip with their sons. They had left for Washington the day before. The team practiced at Centennial Sportsplex that day, and I had Tami take me by there so that I could say hello to some of the fathers that I had become friendly with over the years. They had seen me move around the locker room at the practice rink, barely able to shuffle my feet while holding onto Tami's arm so that I didn't fall.

Kristin called Brandon Walker, the Predators manager of hockey operations, to tell him that the system was turned on and things were working. Brandon told Kristin to get me on videotape. He wanted us to send him something to show the team. They were scheduled to be in a meeting not long after that. Kristin called Tami and told her to get me down to the arena to videotape something.

Tami was driving, Aaron was in the back seat, and I was in the passenger seat. Tami got the phone call from Kristin saying that the team wanted a video to show to the guys. All of a sudden I was half laughing and half crying saying, "I don't know if I can do that."

Tami had never seen me like that and it creeped her out big time. Tami said I didn't have to do it, but I said I wanted to but I didn't know if I could. We made it down to the arena, and I got through taping the piece for the team. At the very end I started to cry, but I did my best to control it. The rest of the day I had the same half laughing, half crying outbursts. It was weird.

The day after the game in Washington, the team practiced at Centennial again. I decided that I was going to try and do a workout, so after practice, I changed into my workout clothes and headed for the treadmill. Trotzy was there in the hallway talking to a couple of members of the media, and kind of like the device inside my body, I turned the treadmill up quickly so that I was basically sprinting on the thing. Trotzy and the reporters that were there stopped what they were doing and were just watching me run really fast. Just two days before, I was in that same building unable to walk on my own.

Through it all, the one thing I never lost was my appetite. I thought I might lose a little weight going through all of this, but I always had a healthy appetite. So in my mind at the time, getting back to working out right away was the smart thing to do.

We didn't know what was going on inside my head. Tami called Dr. Davis the next day and told him that there was something wrong with me. Dr. Davis told her to get me in there. He diagnosed it as emotional lability.

People who have emotional lability, also known as Pseudobulbar affect, have sudden involuntary outbursts of crying or laughing. It was scary going through it, and scary for my family watching me experience it without them being able to understand or do anything for it.

Dr. Davis said they had to turn the system off. They had to change it and go way down. Basically, Dr. Davis had to take it back to zero.

With the cameras around, they took me from 0-60 so that the cameras would be there to capture the seemingly instant results. They thought it was the right thing to do at the time. They are still learning all about it. So instead of 0-60, they had to go 0-10, 10-20 and so on until where I am now, which is where I was when they first did it.

The doctors are brilliant guys and they know right where to put the electrodes and how high to turn it up, but some people can't handle all of the electricity at once, and I was one of those people whose brains couldn't handle it right away.

Right after that, my family said that I was crazy or manic. Soon after the initial emotional lability episode, Tami's dad died and we went to Portland for the services.

I played golf with a few of my buddies in Portland when we were there. I had never sworn before in front of them, and while we were golfing, a string of f-bombs just came out of my mouth one after the other. One of my buddies there said he had heard more curse words come out of me over the course of three holes than he had in all the years he knew me. It was like I had Tourette's syndrome.

After we got back to Nashville, I was spending money left and right and emptied out our checking account. One day I went to a local jewelry store to buy something for Tami. I argued with the saleswoman about the price of a necklace until she finally called the owner of the store. I knew the owner, and he agreed to sell it to me at the price I was looking for because he knew it was for Tami. Another day, I went down to the arena and took Kristin and a bunch of other people from the office out to lunch at The Palm. I didn't know what I was doing.

One day when I was at the office, Barry told me that he needed to talk to me. I said OK, and then immediately started walking upstairs. He started following me upstairs and said; "I guess we are having the meeting upstairs then."

Out of concern for my job, Tami went to David and told him that I was a little bit crazy and not to be offended at what I said to him while we were getting things adjusted. I don't think that I was in any danger of getting fired, but it was nice that she was looking out for me.

Tami lost a bunch of weight in a short period of time worrying about me. We were in Naples, Florida on vacation, and after dinner I went off on a walk. I ended up just sitting on a table down off in some alley talking to some people I just met as I was walking by them. Tami didn't know where I was for about 45 minutes. This is one of those cases where a GPS implanted into the device would have been a great help to my wife.

Tami and the kids would find me all over the house some nights. While in bed, it seemed like every eight seconds I would move my arms or get up and move around. One time, I punched Tami in the head – I tell people I did that one on purpose. Other times they would find me asleep over a chair, on the floor somewhere. Later my doctor gave me a prescription for gabapentin to help control my restless limbs, which were previously controlled by the medications. I didn't even know I had it until I went off of those medications and started hitting Tami while I slept. Now I sleep eight hours through the night, and Tami is safe too.

The mania was a result of us being on the wrong part of the A, B, C, D rod. It was hitting some kind of electron and following a path, so Dr. Davis had to move it away from that part. When he did it, there was a week where I was severely depressed because my right side could not function at all. I was on the road with the team, and both Trotzy and Predators play-by-play announcer Pete Weber called Tami to say there was something wrong with me.

Over time, my brain was able to handle the increased activity. Eventually the manic and crazy episodes went away as the doctors got a better grip on the progression of turning the system up slowly. At that point, Tami stopped feeling that she had to hide the checkbook from me so that that I didn't spend the rest of our money.

Tami did have to hide the external device from me because I wanted more though. They had it set to where I could move it up four or down four. Of course, I would immediately move it up four.

I told Tami that she needed to learn how to work it, but she wasn't into that. Somewhat surprisingly, I talked her into it anyway. We were making adjustments with it one day and Tami accidentally turned it off completely. She said that it was an accident, but I am not sure that I believe her. I actually think that she asked the doctors to place a GPS inside the unit so that she could track me down if she needed to do so.

I was freaking out and Tami said that we needed to get the manual out to figure out how to get it going again.

I said, "I am not looking at the manual."

"OK, we are going to the hospital," she shot back at me.

I told her that I was not going to the hospital. All of a sudden I hit it, and it started back up again. I could tell right away that had kicked back in, so we both won. We didn't have to read the manual or go to the hospital.

Ben Petrick told me that it took about a year after his DBS procedure for them to find his ideal settings. After going through all of that, you would like for them to just flip a switch and have everything be working fine, but everyone is different, it just takes a while. I just had to be patient, something that I am not all that great at doing a lot of times. Now that it is functioning properly, it was definitely worth waiting for.

Every now and then I have bad days and I get frustrated, but it is working like a charm. And Tami is not the only one who has turned the system off on me, Dr. Davis did it to me as well, but it was no accident.

Dr. Davis is a good man. He is really smart. He never gets riled up. He never gets upset or off base. He knows his stuff. He is very calm and he is very good with me because I get a little hyper at times.

One day I went into his office and I was all pissed off that day. I told him that the thing wasn't working. I was bitching and moaning about it. We were about two months after it was activated and I was frustrated. He said let me recalibrate it, but instead of recalibrating it, he turned it completely off to teach me a lesson.

Almost immediately, I started shaking. Tami thought I was faking. She was asking me what I was doing. After a minute, Dr. Davis said, "Oh, I didn't know I had it off."

He turned it back on, and the shaking stopped. He looked at me and said, "This thing does work, doesn't it?"

I said, "OK you are right - now keep it on please!"

If I call him during the day, he calls me back right when he gets back to the office. I couldn't ask for anybody better. When Tami said I was crazy, she called him all of the time. He is a wonderful person. I am a very lucky guy. A lot of doctors are just as smart as Dr. Davis, but his nature and overall bedside manner set him apart from the rest.

He can make you go blind. He can make you see double. He can make you not be able to talk. He taps into certain areas. When we were testing different areas one day, he was trying one thing and my eyes went blurry. Then he tried another thing and I couldn't talk. As time goes on and the Parkinson's progresses, they can adjust the programs. I am going to get bad again, that's just part of it.

Every once in a while, I have pity parties, and sure I feel sorry for myself and I get mad and pissed off, but in the grand scheme of things, I am way better off than a lot of people.

Prior to undergoing DBS, I thought my days of going on golf trips with my friends were over, but just a couple of months after DBS, my golfing group took a trip to TPC Sawgrass during the NHL's All-Star break. One downside to the DBS is that my golf game is horrible now. When the Parkinson's had me all locked up, I had no choice but to keep my arm still. Now that I have free range of motion with my arms, I can't seem to control where the ball goes anymore.

Chapter Twenty-One - Andrew Ference's Stanley Cup Interview

Just minutes after the Boston Bruins won the Stanley Cup in 2010; Scott Oake of the Canadian Broadcasting Company's *Hockey Night in Canada* approached Bruins defenseman Andrew Ference for an interview.

I had the pleasure of coaching Andy in Portland, and he was a member of our Memorial Cup-winning team in 1998. Scott's first question referenced how close Andy came to winning the Stanley Cup with Calgary in 2004, and he named some of his teammates with the Flames who he was thinking of at the time.

Scott's next question was, "Besides former teammates Andrew, who do you think of tonight?"

Andy mentioned how important his parents and sister have been to him throughout his hockey career and his life. Then he paused for a second and said:

"You don't get to this moment without help, and you know what, the one other person other than all of my family members that have supported me so much is Brent Peterson. You know, he was my coach in junior and obviously he is in Nashville now and he has had his own challenges over the last couple of years. There is not a chance that I am here without him. I owe a lot to him."

My family and I were in Florida at the time, so we were not watching CBC's feed of the game and had no idea he had said that about me. In the next few minutes my phone started going crazy with calls, text messages, and emails from all of my friends and family in Canada asking me if I saw the interview.

When I did see it, I was just floored. It brought tears to my eyes. I hadn't coached the guy since 1998 and I was one of the first people he thought of after winning hockey's most cherished prize.

Moments like that make everything I have ever gone through over the years worth it. Just knowing that I made enough of a difference in a kid's life to carry that with him into adulthood is staggering.

Andy called me the week after my Parkinson's diagnosis became public. He told me that if I ever needed anything from him at any time to not hesitate to call him, and he meant it. That is the kind of guy he is. Even though we never see each other outside of once a year or so when our teams play each other, he has never forgotten me. We still talk on the phone every so often.

When Andy was having his day with the Stanley Cup, he called me and told me that he wanted me to be there with him. I didn't get the call directly, but he left me a nice voicemail message. I returned his call a couple of days later, and when he picked up, there was a lot of noise in the background. I asked him what was going on and he told me that he was on the float and that their Stanley Cup parade was about to start. Seriously, the guy took my call as he was about to parade through the streets of Boston to celebrate with literally a million Bruins fans. He is an amazing guy.

His day with the Cup was in Boston in September before the 2011-12 season started. I was not doing all that well physically at the time, and it was a couple of days before my golf tournament and party, so I was not able to go up to Boston to spend the day with him. Just getting the invite was touching though.

Andy is a small defensive-defenseman, but he gets every bit out of his play. He just plays hard every single shift, every single day whether it is in games or in practice. He is just a tough, tough kid. We got him in Portland when he was 15-years-old and we as a coaching staff said, "Wow, he is the best player on the ice for us." And that was with Andy going up against kids that were up to 20-years-old. That is a huge gap at that age, but he handled it. He is a great player with a strong grasp of the game.

A year before Andy won the Cup, Marian Hossa, another one of the players on the Memorial Cup team from Portland, won the Stanley Cup with the Chicago Blackhawks. Once I was somewhat over the fact that we were the ones Chicago knocked out of the first round of the playoffs, I was rooting for Hossa to win that Cup. Marian and Andy were two guys who I really wanted to win Stanley Cups, and they did it in back-to-back seasons.

Right when he got to Portland, I knew Hossa was going to make it. He was a terrific kid. He came to us with big accolades, but he was very respectful and wasn't a big shot. If I sat him down because he wasn't playing well, he just took it and played harder. He knew English when he came over from Slovakia, so I think that helped his transition to North America and the North American style of hockey immensely.

To this day, when he plays a game in Nashville, he always searches out my wife to see her and talk to her for a little while. He is just a class guy and a world-class hockey player.

As happy as I was for Andy and Marian to win their Stanley Cups, now it is time for the Nashville Predators to win one. David Poile, Trotzy, Peter Horachek, and I have all worked too hard over the years not to get one. Ever since I entered the NHL as a player, that has been my goal, and that goal has not changed. I may not be able to coach any longer, but I know that I can still help this team win one. The Stanley Cup is why we play the game. It is the ultimate goal whether you are a player, coach, manager, equipment guy, or anyone else associated with an NHL team.

As much as I want to win it personally and for the other coaches and David, I really want to bring the Stanley Cup here to Nashville for the fans. We have a dedicated group of fans that has stuck with us over the years. There have been times where it has not been easy to be a fan of the Predators. The early years were very lean. We did not have a big budget and therefore did not have a lot of talented players. When some of our players became good, we no longer had the ability to afford to keep them, so they ended up going to other teams. Our fans have also survived two lockouts as well as a near hostile takeover by BlackBerry guru Jim Balsillie. He wanted to buy the team and move it to Hamilton, Ontario.

Our new ownership group has stabilized things, and our product on the ice has been good. Our fans have responded by packing Bridgestone Arena for our home games and given us an amazing amount of support in our pursuit of the Cup.

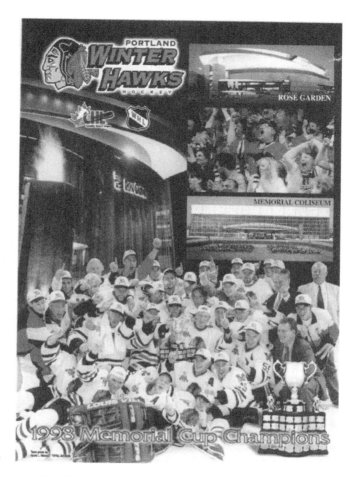

The 1998 Memorial Cup championship celebration
(Portland Winterhawks)

Chapter Twenty-Two - Advisor, Not Coach

As much as DBS has given me, the one thing that it has not done for me is given me the chance to be a hockey coach again.

The one thing that DBS does not correct is balance. I fall down all the time, and that is just when I stand up or I am walking around. If I bang my head from falling when I am just waking around, I could do some serious damage trying to be out on the ice again.

That means I can never go back out on the ice. A coach, especially an assistant or an associate head coach, needs to be on the ice with the players. Before practice, after practice, at the morning skates, those are the times that the assistants get the quality one-on-one time with the players when it is most needed. I can't do that, so I can never coach again.

Every once in a while I feel sorry for myself as I see these different guys getting coaching jobs in the NHL and I think that I am a better coach than they are. There are guys who fail in one place just to go on and get another job somewhere else. I know that I could have been a head coach in the NHL, and I know that if I was given the opportunity I would have done well.

I am done forever as far as coaching is concerned because I can't do the job full-time. I am glad that the Predators have kept me on as a hockey operations advisor though. Sure I get locked up and I can't do some things, but I am not nearly as bad off as some people are. I can still work, be productive, and help the organization out in a lot of ways.

I joke with Trotzy and David sometimes that now I am in the position of being an advisor I can never be wrong. If I tell them something and they take my advice and it works, I look like a genius. If I tell them something and they think to themselves – "Ah, Petey is crazy," don't do what I tell them, do things their way and it backfires, I still look like a genius and they look silly for not listening to me. Really, it is a no lose situation for me.

Being an advisor is good, but if you get too many people in your ear, it clouds the issue. Trotzy trusts me, but he also has David, Peter and Lane giving him advice. He has to rely on his assistant coaches, but I can come in and help at certain times and advise on certain things.

When I was coaching, I knew what I wanted. I had to go out and had to go by feel of who should be on the ice. You can't sit up in the press box and second-guess the coaches. "You need to have this guy out there, or that guy out there," well maybe there is a reason that guy wasn't out there. When Suter and Weber were young, I didn't have them out there all the time. There were reasons why I had them out there or didn't have them on the ice. I knew what I was doing. Sometimes having too many voices can cause problems. Too many voices can cause indecision. I am not there all day, every day with the players, so they have to make their own decisions and I would never second-guess them.

I can give my opinion before the game, but I can't go and tell Peter and those guys much late in the third period. When the game is on the line, they have to feel how things are going from down at ice level. During the game and at the intermissions, coaches will get feedback from players about how things are going on the ice. I just don't have that feel or connection sitting upstairs.

After people had seen me since undergoing DBS, there have been some inquiries as to whether or not I was interested in making a return to coaching.

I thought about it for a while, but I realized that I couldn't do it. At some point I am going to get bad again. It is a short-term thing to think I can coach, but it is not a reality. My tenure is over. I know that. I could probably do it for a month or half of a season, but I know that eventually it would catch up to me. Coaches have such long hours and such tough jobs; there is just no way I can do it anymore. I just have to learn how to accept it. I could go behind the bench, but you have to be able to build relationships with players, talking to them before practice, after practice. That is what I was good at doing. The coaches that do that are successful, the ones that don't are not.

The reality is that my coaching days have ended. There is, unfortunately, no way I can pursue my dream.

I am a good advisor. I know when to get in and when to get out of David or Trotzy's ears. I am going to have to be semi-retired. I am not a full-time person anymore.

I could never leave Nashville now. I am a Predator for life.

Chapter Twenty-Three - My Coaching Philosophy

I have always believed that if you build good relationships with your players, especially the core group of players, that is a recipe for success. I built relationships with them because we had to go through tough times together. Of course there were times that I had to come down hard on my players. When I did, they knew that I had their backs and they had mine as well. You want to get to know them as much as they want to get to know you. Then when you do have a bad stretch and have to come down hard on them, everyone knows that we all can get through it together.

Everybody has a different philosophy. Some guys don't want to have any kind of relationship with their players so that they can just get rid of them when they need to and not feel it emotionally. I think that is for the short-term guys. Guys like that don't seem to last too long in one place. Long-term guys are honest — like Trotzy, he is a long-term guy, he works hard, and he prepares his players. His message is the same, but he just changes it around a little every year.

There needs to be some separation there, but you can't always have an "us against them" or a "them against us" mentality. There has to be some 'we' togetherness. Most coaches are pretty good guys and they just want to win. There has never been one player who I have had that I disliked them as a person. There were some that I disliked as a player, but you have to make that separation.

The reason that some coaches do not want to get to know their players is that they have to make decisions that will hurt them as a person and they don't want to feel attached. If you are a good coach, you can get to know them and still make decisions about them. You have to. There are some guys you just have to let go of at times. You have to move on and do the right thing for the team. There are certain players that will always say, "The coaches didn't like me."

This may not come as a big surprise to people, but coaches like winning. One thing they don't like is getting fired. Winning games helps coaches keep their jobs. It is a pretty simple formula.

If I didn't get to know my players on a personal level, I think that I would have gone crazy. If you can't get along with your players, who can you get along with? You are with them every day for up to eight months. You can't just develop a relationship over a short period of time, it has to be done over a long period.

One summer early in his professional career, I went up to Wisconsin and I got to know Ryan Suter very well away from the ice. Another time I went over to Europe and met some guys. The guys I met over there, I became friends with – like Kimmo Timonen for example. I met him in Finland, and got to know him there. That extra effort of going to talk with them in their hometowns of their home countries really meant a lot to them. If I build a relationship with a player and he doesn't do a certain thing, I can go to him and say, "This is what is best for you and what you have to do." If he doesn't like that, he still knows that I am a normal guy and I have a family.

Some guys just think that you are a guy way up here and he can't talk to you, but that is not the way it is.

You are a coach and you tell them that they have to work out and do this and that to get by. You can't survive if you can't do that. You have to first build a relationship with your players. That's what I was going to do if I ever became a head coach. I was going to visit every guy that I could the first summer and try to see them in their environment and find out what they are made of – what pushes their buttons, whether they need a kick in the pants or whether you need to put your arm around them, whatever it takes to motivate them.

Coaches may just not like the way a player plays. It has nothing to do with us as coaches not liking them. If we didn't like what they did on the ice, that's when you had to make a decision that was best for the team. If a coach makes a decision for the team, it is for the best of the team, if a guy wasn't a part of it, that's just the way it was.

If one of those decisions is made, you just have to tell them that the other guy just came in and played better than you. It was not about us screwing them over because we didn't like them as a person. That's a farce. If a player was bad off of the ice, I had no time for him at all.

You can only be a complete idiot ranting and raving for so long. That only works for a little while. And it doesn't even work on everybody in the short term. You just say you have to play harder or you don't play. Positive things are way better than being negative all the time. I just don't think you have to be that way. Every once in a while you have to yell at the guys and say something funny like, "You are going to drive me to drink if you don't get going."

When I was interviewing for the head coaching job in Vancouver, I called some of the other GMs around the league to find out what they wanted from different people.

I called Brian Burke one day, and he said, "Petey, I really like you as a person, but I would never hire you as a head coach."

I said, "What are you talking about?"

"You are too nice," he said. "I can't have a nice coach."

To me, that is shortsightedness. I don't think that works in the long run. I am not Mr. Nice Guy. If I have to make a decision on a player, I am not afraid of making that decision, but I don't have to treat them cruelly.

You want to be fair and honest, that's all that you can be. It is being logical.

You treat all of the players differently, but I tried to be equally fair with all of them. Some players are very skilled and earn a lot of ice time. The salaries the players get these days are all over the place, but that can't have any bearing on how fairly they are treated.

Some players just need to be talked to differently than the others.

In Portland, I had a guy named Adam Deadmarsh, and I had to make him mad at me and kick him in the butt. When I did that, he would go out there and work harder. Other guys needed to be stroked and they couldn't be yelled at in front of anybody else or else I would lose them. Adam, I could do anything to him and he would get madder at me and go out and kick somebody's butt that night. That's the way he was wired. Everybody has a different button to push. If they are at that level, they are good enough to play, and they will be good somehow. Some guys just can't find the motivation to play every night, and that's your job as a coach to try to get them to play the same every game – to the best of their abilities. Whatever you can do to talk to them or piss them off, it will make better players and better team players.

You know right away what guys are going to be NHL guys. Some make it that you don't think and some that should make it don't make it. Deadmarsh was a good player, but he was a great NHLer because he just played hard.

Some guys need some guidance. Other guys don't know how to lead. Some guys make everybody else around them better, others don't. It is just a matter of how you want to do it. Usually if you pick the right players, and you do things the right way, you will build a good team.

I would have no problem bringing in any young center to watch Mike Fisher in how he plays and how he acts off of the ice. There are other players I wouldn't want younger guys to be around off of the ice. It is just a matter of who your mentors are.

Players need to motivate themselves. They need to find good guys to follow. If they follow guys like Fisher or Shea Weber, they are going to find out how to become good pros.

Some guys separate themselves from all of the others. Some guys get their money and sort of float until they have to do it again the next time their contract comes up for renewal. Most guys that have any kind of character play hard all the time no matter what. Those are the guys I always wanted on my team, and those are the kinds of guys I will always push for in the future.

In the NHL, there are a bunch of players who are just good. There are some bad players that are playing too. The ones who have character and are good are superstars. The ones who have no skill at all but have character can get by. The ones that have lots of skill and no character, they don't last very long. Once you have character and you have work ethic and you have skill, then you have a superstar. That's just the way it is. The cream always rises to the top. I know it is cliché, but it is true.

If we send a guy down to the minors and he does the job down there, we will notice him and he will be back. If he doesn't, we will notice that too. You want to see how he does down in the minors. The guys that do well down there will find a way to get it done. We don't care who is up here, we just care that the guy that is up here does the job.

Being an assistant is a different job than a head coach. The head coach has to have a grip on motivating the players and handling the media. Assistant coaches can handle all of the Xs and Os. When you are comfortable in your own skin, you can do anything you want. I think the best way is to be honest and upstanding and treat people the right way.

I tried to take a lot of the lessons I learned during my playing career and apply them to my players when I was coaching.

Just about all of the junior and college players who get drafted all put up big offensive numbers when they were younger, but when they get to the NHL, everyone they are playing against are stars on both the offensive and defensive ends of the ice.

When I got into the league, I was a lot like Nick Spaling who plays for the Predators now. In juniors he had great offensive statistics, but when he got to the NHL, we needed him to do more than try and score.

I had to learn to take faceoffs when I got to the NHL. Going in, I wasn't any better at taking draws than anybody else. I didn't really care much about it to tell you the truth. I quickly realized that I had to learn how to check and how to be a good penalty killer if I was planning on staying in the NHL for any length of time at all.

When I got to Buffalo, Craig Ramsay taught me how to play a solid two-way game. He used to get mad at me because I never tried to score. He told me, "You are still a good player. You have to go score. You can't just sit back and be a defensive player."

That is what I tried to tell my guys, and to some degree, I still do it as part of my role as an advisor. Two-way players are way more valuable than a guy that can only check or a guy that can only score and doesn't work hard on the defensive end. You are a valuable player if you work hard, two-ways, take the body, and do those things. Those are some good lessons, some tough lessons, some good times and some tough times.

The whole game is about winning. It is not about one guy making a lot of money. 50 goals don't do anything if they don't help you win. That's what Scotty Bowman taught Steve Yzerman in Detroit. Early in his career he had 50 goals every year, but they didn't win anything. Scotty told him to play a little defense, play some two-way hockey. Scotty told him that his goal totals would come down a little, but the team will win. Sure enough, Yzerman did what Scotty told him to do and they won. Now Yzerman is looked at as one of the best captains in the history of the league. He is the general manager of the Tampa Bay Lightning, and you can be sure that he is having his coaching staff teach the players to play the way Scotty taught him to do it.

Chapter Twenty-Four - The Birth of a Foundation

After I was diagnosed with Parkinson's, my good friend Peter Jacobsen kept talking to me about starting a foundation to try and raise money for Parkinson's research. Being a professional golfer, Peter knew that having my name attached to something would be a good way to go about raising money.

For a few years, I didn't really want to have anything to do with that.

Then one day after taking the dog for a walk, I came into the house and heard just the craziest thing. I couldn't believe my ears. Tami had the TV on, and someone was replaying a portion of Rush Limbaugh's radio show from that day. Limbaugh was attacking Michael J. Fox for a political ad he had taped for a candidate for political office in Missouri. Michael was supporting that candidate because she was for stem cell research, and he was hopeful that the stem cell research would help Parkinson's patients.

During his radio show, Limbaugh basically called Michael a liar. During the ad, Michael was having pretty severe tremors, and Limbaugh said that he was faking it. It was even to the point that Limbaugh was moving around in his chair imitating Michael's movements. He said that Michael must not have taken his medication the day that they filmed the ad.

That was the defining moment for me. To no one in particular, I said, "He is not faking it. I know that I am not faking it."

That was it. That was when I knew that I had to do something to help raise awareness and raise some money to help people with Parkinson's. It took five years, but that was enough to get me off of my butt.

Soon thereafter, I got on the board of the American Parkinson's Disease Association. That is when we decided to do our first golf tournament. We had a little golf tournament and we raised somewhere between $25 and 30 thousand for Parkinson's research. The only problem was that the money went to APDA. We didn't know where the money went. I think that only about $5,000 went to Michael J. Fox's foundation, but we had no control over the rest of it.

I did all of this work and I didn't know where the money went or have any control over it. That was when I decided to organize Peterson for Parkinson's.

Along with some of my good friends here in Nashville, we put a board together and the foundation became a reality. We kept the golf tournament as our major fundraiser, and now all of the money is in the control of the foundation and the board decides where it goes.

The foundation's board of directors is great. They aren't a bunch of yes men and women. If I have a good idea, they tell me that. If I have a crazy idea, they aren't afraid to tell me that too. They really give it to me if I don't do something right. They really push me to be better, to do the right things to raise awareness.

After a couple of years of just having the golf tournament, I decided that we would have a dinner the night before as well. It was for the golfers and people who weren't going to golf, but wanted to help PFP out in another way. We do everything first-class at the dinners; good food and drink, some great entertainment, and some really interesting silent auction items. I am a firm believer that doing things in a first-class manner is the way to go. It may cost a little more to put them on this way, but I think that it is a big incentive to people to keep coming back year after year.

All of the teams from around the NHL have been great about helping us out with items for the silent auctions. Every year, we have jerseys from all of the top stars in the league like Sidney Crosby and Alex Ovechkin, not to mention all kinds of items from the Predators.

We try to split the dinner into some entertaining parts, and some educational parts as well. One year, Dr. Davis and Dr. Bowman got up and spoke about Parkinson's and the research they are doing at Vanderbilt. They were great at talking to the crowd in terms that everyone could understand. Their enthusiasm for the progress that they have made in research really got the crowd motivated. It was easy to tell that the people there were happy to be a part of something that has the potential to positively impact the lives of so many that have Parkinson's.

We have also had comedians and magicians perform at the dinners. There has also been a surprise guest or two make an appearance.

In February of 2011, the Predators acquired Mike Fisher in a trade with the Ottawa Senators. Mike's wife Carrie Underwood is rather famous, especially in Nashville.

The day of the trade, the local paper's headline was "Predators trade for Carrie Underwood's husband." The people in Canada got a lot of run out of that one.

Prior to that summer's dinner, Carrie agreed to appear and sing a song. I made sure not to tell anyone so that it was a surprise to all. When it came time for her to sing, I told the crowd that we had a special guest that night and then introduced "Mike Fisher's wife" onto the stage. When she came up, she gave me a kiss on the cheek. After she did that, I stammered my words a little and acted a little dumb. Tami says that I wasn't acting, but in reality, I was.

Carrie brought her guitarist up with her and they did a beautiful song. It was amazing. We had almost 1,000 people in Bridgestone Arena that night, and at least half of them had their smartphones out recording the performance.

Later that night, we turned one of the silent auction items into a live auction. It was the night's big prize, a trip for two with the Predators on a four-game trip out west. The winner of the auction got to go on the team's charter plane, ride the busses with the team, stay in the team hotel, and tickets to the games. We put the value on this item as priceless because these opportunities just don't present themselves very often if at all.

We started with the last bid on the trip from the silent auction and tried to run it up higher. I served as the auctioneer. Really, there is no end to the number of talents that I possess.

With all of the bright lights that were focused on the stage, I could not see a whole lot. There were a few more bids, but then it was just Carrie and some other guy from farther off of the stage. I could not see him at all.

When Carrie kept bidding, I looked over at Mike and said, "Fish, your wife can't come on the charter with the team."

When it appeared that neither Carrie nor the other guy were going to back down from the other, I quickly decided that four people were going to go on that trip if we could just agree on a price and let both of them win it. That is what happened. Oh, and Carrie did not come on the trip, she was nice enough to give it to Mike's brothers so they came with us out west.

But the big sellers at the dinners are Petey's Balls. Each year, we get 100 numbered golf balls and sell each numbered ball for $100. They are affectionately known as Petey's Balls. At the end of the night, we reveal the prizes associated with each numbered ball. Everyone gets a prize worth at least $100, but we also have some prizes that are worth a whole lot more.

The balls sell out very quickly. I always have a good time when I go on radio shows promoting the golf tournament and dinner. I love making the hosts squirm by talking about the popularity of Petey's Balls and that people need to get to the dinners early if they want to get their hands on one of Petey's Balls. I don't think that any of the hosts have had to hit the dump button on me yet. I make sure to have fun with it, but not to the point where the Federal Communications Commission will step in and fine the radio station for any kind of indecency violations.

The idea to have the dinner the night before the golf tournament turned out to be a great one. The first two years we had the dinners, we held them at the Factory in Franklin, but we quickly outgrew that space and now it is held at Bridgestone Arena.

In 2011, we decided to combine forces with the Nashville Predators Foundation for the golf tournament and party. In prior years, we would have a golf tournament and the Predators Foundation would have one about a week later.

The golf tournaments are always fun, but they are a lot of work and there are many challenges. We are usually great about adjusting on the fly to whatever challenge is presented to us though.

After the 2011 tournament I saw a group of guys coming off of the course.

I went up to them to thank them for playing. After some small talk, I asked them which celebrity played with them that day.

"Our celebrity didn't show up today," one of them said.

There is always one celebrity that forgets about the tournament or has travel problems and can't get into Nashville in time. I just happened to find that one group this day. I did not want them to have a bad experience or impression of the tournament that carries my name, so I wanted to try and make it right with them.

I told them that we would find a day that the Predators were playing in Nashville and go golfing together at Legends that morning. I told them that I would take them to dinner before the game and if the Predators won the game that night, I would bring them down to the locker room and have them meet all the players.

After I outlined all of that, I asked them if that would make up for their celebrity not showing up that day, and they assured me that it would. As I was walking away, one of them stopped me.

"Hey coach, when we sign up for next year's tournament, can you make sure that our celebrity doesn't show up then either? We really like the idea of getting all of that extra stuff."

Crisis averted – they obviously were good with how I wanted to make it up to them, even to the point of joking with me about it.

We have other satellite golf tournaments now. Starting in 2010, we have one in Fenelon Falls, Ontario started by great friends Phil and Lori Baker, and another one started in Edmonton in 2012. I spend time going to them and getting to know the people who are raising money on behalf of the foundation.

People have been so generous about giving to PFP and taking it upon themselves to raise money for it. For the last couple of years, several people who have run the Country Music Marathon and Half Marathon have gone out and solicited donations from their friends and families to sponsor them running on behalf of PFP. This has been really successful for the foundation. We have everything set up on our website so that people can just go there and pick out the runner that they wish to sponsor.

We set the runners up with PFP shirts to wear during the race. That way, people who see them out on the course can ask them about the foundation if they are unfamiliar with it. And hey, running with Team Petey on their shirts has to be a motivator all on its own.

It is not easy asking people for money, especially in a down economy, but I know that I am doing the right thing in raising funds through the foundation. We give most of the money raised to Vanderbilt for the research they are doing right here in Nashville. That money goes into a special fund so they can show us exactly what they do with it. I have been there so many times and seen the direct benefits of the money we have given to them over the years. It is so motivating to know that I have had some kind of an impact into the research that is being done on this horrible disease.

Not all of the money we collect goes to research though, as we also give some directly to programs that serve Parkinson's patients.

We try to help the caregivers as well.

Caregivers are so important. When I see what my wife had to go through, I know what other people have to go through each and every day. They are the forgotten people in all of this. Everybody feels sorry for me, but no one knows what Tami had to go through over the years. I feel great compared to most people. I am fortunate that I have been able to do this.

I am grateful that the Predators have kept me on so that I can still do my work with the team, but work with the foundation as well. They take great care of me.

Not only has the team allowed me to keep a job, they have been so generous financially too. The players all show up to the dinners and the golf tournaments. David Poile has generously given to the foundation for each goal the team scores during the season. This disease is one that is very familiar to him, since his father Bud Poile was afflicted with it. The ownership group has also given the foundation a lot of money. In 2011, Joel Dobberphul, one of the owners, pledged a dollar for every mile flown during the playoffs. We made two round trips from Nashville to Anaheim and Vancouver that year, so those miles translated into a lot of money. They presented me with a large check at that year's foundation dinner. It is just staggering how many people are so giving.

In 2012, we set it up on the website where anyone could pledge on a per mile basis; whether it was a dollar or a penny. It may be cliché, but everything helps us in our quest to educate and raise awareness about Parkinson's.

None of this would be possible without the amazing people that so graciously sit on the Board of PFP.

Deb Lowenthal has been a great friend all of these years and she has run my foundation as the executive director since we started it.

The board members are: Amy Breedlove, Lynn and Kay Ellsworth, John and Barbara Holmes, John and Valerie Overmyer, Gavenn and Ramona Ross, Candace Price, Jay Lowenthal, Phil Baker, Bret Fincher, Peter Jacobsen, Chris Stout, Barry Trotz, Peter Horachek, and Tami Peterson.

All of them have been terrific, and PFP is successful thanks to all of the hard work they have put in through the years. There is no way I can thank them enough for all they have done for the foundation and for me personally.

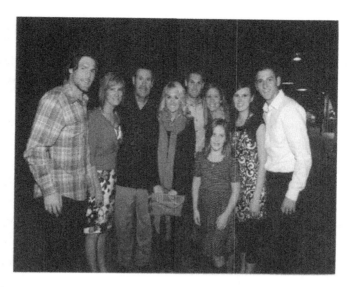

The Peterson Family with Mike Fisher and Carrie Underwood at the 2011
Peterson for Parkinson's Foundation dinner (Peterson Family Photo)

Chapter Twenty-Five - Life Coach

In addition to my role with the Predators and working with my foundation, I have also been fortunate to be a life coach for others who have been diagnosed with Parkinson's.

A few years ago, a friend of mine who used to work for the Portland Trail Blazers called me and told me that a guy by the name of Brian Grant had recently been diagnosed with Parkinson's and was not dealing with it very well. Brian was still in his 30s and had recently retired from the NBA. It had been about six months since his diagnosis, and I knew exactly what he was going through.

I told my friend that I was going to be in Portland visiting my in-laws, so I would be happy to talk to Brian and try and help him in any way that I possibly could. We met at a tiny little restaurant where Brian liked to eat, right down on the river in Portland. He came in and sat slumped over at the table. He listened to me tell my story for about an hour.

All he would say was, "This is not fair. I don't deserve this, I'm too young…" and on and on. So, I basically gave him the same speech that Michael J. Fox gave to me and told him that you can continue to act like this or you can go do something about it.

He said he couldn't do what I was doing. He didn't want to have a golf tournament or have a foundation. I told him that everybody in Portland loves him and that he was a great guy. I told him that trying to go through this alone was not the way to do it.

It took a couple of hours, but I finally convinced him that he could do something about it. He got some people together and they put together a great foundation. He went to Phoenix and met Muhammad Ali and brought him in for his golf tournament. He went and met Michael J. Fox and piggybacked with MJF and made over $300,000 in two days for the MJF foundation. I went to the event as well. It was a great feeling because he did something about it after initially not wanting to do anything or deal with anyone.

That next year, he came to our event because I was there for him, so he said that he wanted to be there to support my foundation and me. Brian had a great time. He got along with the players. Even though he said that he didn't want to speak,

I pressured him into it and he did a great job.

Brian was sitting at the table with Tami and everyone else who spoke that night.

He told Tami, "I'm not going up there." Tami had to rub his back and tell him, "You will do great." He got up there and he was fantastic. He captivated the audience. Although he is 6'9" and a hulking physical presence, he is so soft-spoken and so down to earth that it seemed like he was a natural public speaker.

Brian told the audience about his foundation and everyone got a good laugh when he told him that the name of his foundation was Shake It Till We Make It.

I think it is great that Brian had a sense of humor when finding a name for his foundation. He has tremors, and everyone who is around him can see that. By acknowledging that fact in the name of his foundation, it puts people at ease somewhat. They can talk to him about it without feeling too uncomfortable.

At the end of Brian's speech, he looked directly at the audience and said, "You guys will find us a cure so that one day I can go to my kids, my two daughters and say, 'They found a cure.'"

That brought everyone to his or her feet. That is a pretty good result for a guy who did not want to get up and speak. He was great. After he spoke, he was talking to a reporter and said that when he played basketball, he thought of himself as a warrior and that when I was talking to him, he recognized that warrior spirit in me.

I didn't think that I had a warrior spirit, but who am I to argue with that?

When talking with other Parkinson's patients I am not all that nice about it. I can't sit there and hold their hand and tell them that everything is going to be fine. It is not going to be fine. This is a horrible disease and they are headed down a long and difficult road. I have been down that road, so they know that I am speaking from a place of experience. A good dose of reality may just be what they need to get out of the stage where they are constantly feeling sorry for themselves.

Anytime I hear of someone who is diagnosed with Parkinson's, I try to reach out to him or her. Some have not wanted to talk to me while others have. It all depends on where they are mentally at the time. There have been some other athletes and coaches who have Parkinson's, some who have come forward with their diagnosis while others have not yet done so for a variety of reasons. Just letting people know that there is a resource available to them is important. I want to let them know that I am available to talk with them if they ever need someone who has been through what they are dealing with every day.

Chapter Twenty-Six - Great Friends

I have some great friends who are nothing but first class people who give of themselves no matter what. I know that if I need them; they are going to be there for me.

When things were really bad, I found out how many great friends I really had.

There are amazingly good people in hockey. It is gratifying being a coach. The players are not getting in trouble off the ice. They are helping people and doing good things for others. People don't understand how good our guys are. You don't find better people than people in hockey.

When I was traded to Buffalo from Detroit, I had four really close friends. Craig Ramsay was my hockey mentor. He taught me everything about the game. Mike Ramsey, Larry Playfair and Lindy Ruff were terrific close friends as well. After our playing careers were over, we all became coaches and have all done very well.

When I went to Hartford, Ray Ferraro and I became good friends. We used to drive to the rink together every day.

A hockey locker room can be one of the most ruthless places known to man. The guys can really get on each other about anything and everything, so it helps to have thick skin. A few years ago, the *Nashville City Paper* did a story about my battle with Parkinson's. They had a picture of me on the cover of the paper that day. One of the players managed to get their hands on about 50 copies of the paper and cut out the cover and taped all of the pictures of my face all over the locker room at the practice facility at Centennial Sportsplex.

They all had a big laugh over it, and in reality, it is just the way hockey players treat those that are close to them. If they didn't care about me, they wouldn't have even bothered doing something like that.

I still told them all that they were a bunch of jerks for making fun of the disabled guy. There was no way that I was going to let them get the last word in on the subject.

The players, other coaches, and management staff of the Predators have all become good friends.

There really is a family atmosphere in the organization.

Since the first time I met Trotzy, he has been the most loyal, honest great friend for all of these years. Peter Horachek has become a great friend and now Lane Lambert has too. David Poile has been a great friend as well. We trust each other and lean on each other for all of these things all these years.

When I was in Portland, Mike Williamson was my assistant coach. He was one of my players and my captain and then he became my assistant coach. He has been a true friend ever since then.

In February 2012, I was inducted into the Hall of Fame in Portland and a lot of my former players came back for the ceremony. To have them come back on a night when I was being honored was a very special feeling.

John Holmes, John Overmyer, and Lynn Ellsworth are the friends who go on golf trips with me. We have been to Pinehurst, Sawgrass, Pumpkin Ridge, Bandon Dunes and many other great courses. They are members of PFP's Board of Directors. They work hard as members of the board, and it is great to be able to travel and spend time with them playing golf, something we all love doing.

Players like Jerred Smithson and Scott Nichol were two guys who I became particularly close with when they played for me. These guys were faceoff guys and penalty killers. Since I was responsible for coaching these units, we spent a lot of time together.

Since their roles were just like I had when I was a player, I just knew where they were coming from. No matter what they did, they never got any glory. They did their jobs. They had a dirty job to do. Sometimes management wouldn't appreciate their roles and they wouldn't get all of the accolades and certainly weren't paid as much as the rest of the other players. They are the ones that blocked the shots and took pucks in the face and did all of those things. That's the way I was, and it is safe to say that I have a special place in my heart for guys like that.

Scotty played for me in Portland and later for the Predators. A lot of people would tease him and call him my other son. That was pretty funny. He is a great person.

Most of those kinds of guys have become coaches and teachers of young men, instructing them about how to become good people and good hockey players. The stars usually don't do that because 1. They have the money and 2. They don't have to do it.

Teaching and coaching are hard jobs. Coaches are like teachers. Teachers don't get paid anything for the jobs they do. Head coaches are starting to get paid, but a lot of the assistant coaches are the ones that teach and do a lot of the work. If you have good assistant coaches that teach your guys, they are examples to them. You have to bring in good guys that are examples to your younger guys. If you tell them that they have to do this, and this, and this, and he doesn't do it, the other guys will ask why doesn't he do it? We want someone who is going to teach the young guys and be an example for them so that those younger players will become good professionals and good players.

One bad egg can spoil the whole locker room. I want guys who play hard every night and skate their legs off, go to the net, and get cross-checked. If some other guy doesn't even work hard coming back, I know he is talented, but it is not fair and I don't want a guy like that on my team.

Once I turned into a coach, I hated to do a kind of defensive system. I wanted to go for it and go balls to the wall to get something happening. That is the way you want to coach. Every year, they had to prove themselves to the coach. I know what they were going through because I had to do it every year. I never had a moment to relax. I always had to be on guard for my job because some kid or some free agent was coming along to take it. Sooner or later your time is over there and you go on to the next place.

Off the ice, a lot of people away from hockey have become good friends too. All of the people on my Board have done so much for me and for the foundation too.

We wouldn't want to live anywhere else, mainly because of all the friends we have here in Nashville. We have friends in other areas, but the people here have been terrific for me. I choke up every time I think about how lucky I am to have all of these people in my life. If I didn't have them, I couldn't get by.

Over the last couple of years, I have had to say goodbye to some friends who passed on way too early.

Late in the summer of 2011, Wade Belak died tragically. He had just ended his playing career and was transitioning into a broadcasting role with the Predators.

Not long after Wade passed away, my good friend Mike Heimerdinger did as well.

Mike and I met one morning at Legends Golf Club. He had just come into town and I had been here for a few years. He told me that he was working for the Titans. I told him that I worked for the Predators. He said that he was their offensive coordinator and I told him I was a defensive coordinator of sorts.

We started playing golf together in the mornings. One day he got there five minutes before I did, so the next day, I made sure that I got there five minutes earlier than he did. Then it was like back and forth until one day when we both pulled into the parking lot at about ten minutes until six. It was pitch dark, and he looked at me and said, "We are sick puppies, aren't we?" Our tee time was not until 7:00 that day. We were both competitive guys and we were even trying to beat each other to the course.

Dinger was very good to me. Then Titans head coach Jeff Fisher became good friends with Barry and me. We went down on the field one day for an exhibition game and the guys told us to stay back when there was a punt. The guys came running down the field and got pushed out of bounds and then went running right back in bounds. It was wild. We went in and did the coin toss. It was just an exhibition game, so they let me pick the coin toss.

We went to visit Dinger down at the Titans headquarters and he showed us around and all of the different things they did with their headsets during the games. We took some of the things we learned from them and used them during our games. Our practices are very scheduled and theirs are always done very last minute. We learned a lot from Jeff and Dinger and they became very good friends.

He came golfing with us one day and said his back was sore. He went in and got an MRI and that is when they found a big lump in his back. It spread all over, and finally they told him that they couldn't do anything more for him. He looked all over for help. He was a tough guy. He worked hard.

One Friday night I got a call. I was in Carolina with the team, and it was Jeff calling me with the bad news. He said, "Petey, it doesn't look like Dinger is going to make it."

Dinger was in Mexico at the time. He had gone all over the world trying to find alternative treatments as an effort to treat his cancer. They helped him for a little while, but his body just had cancer everywhere. He was in Mexico and someone tried to send a plane to get him, but he died before they could get him out, and he had to stay there for a little bit. The next week we had the funeral. It was tough.

Two other deaths have had a significant impact upon my life. Tami has a very close-knit family. Just before Christmas in 2006, Tami received a devastating phone call with the news that her only brother Ty, two years older than she, had passed away in his sleep at the age of 49, suffering from cardiac arrest. It was a terrible shock to the whole family. My schedule allowed me to make the trip to Portland to participate in his funeral. He was quite a character and we celebrated his life with many stories. He was a writer by profession but had multiple talents including music. One of his students was Tommy Thayer of "Kiss" who Ty had taught to play the guitar.

In January of 2012, following years of dealing with dementia, Tami's father Ralph was allowed to move on from this life. We knew it was coming, but still, the loss was difficult. He slipped away 15 minutes before we arrived in Portland.

Tami and her sister Suzi put together a beautiful service, and even though I was just out of DBS surgery, I participated again. We were overwhelmed with the many floral arrangement from our Predators family and other Tennessee friends that arrived at the church.

It was sad to see my good friends and family members go. Through all of that, I have learned how precious life is and how quickly it can end.

Chapter Twenty-Seven - Looking Ahead

DBS was a very long and very involved process, but now that I have completed the process and the system is functioning as it should, I realize that I have been given a very special gift, the gift of time.

The way my Parkinson's was progressing prior to DBS, it did not look like I had a whole lot of quality time left. I was locked up more often and for longer periods of time, and since the disease is a progressive one, there is no doubt that it would have continued along that road.

Now that I am feeling better, I have been given a second chance and I intend to do the most with it. Both personally and professionally I still have a lot that I want to accomplish.

I cherish the time I spend with my family and friends.

I still love coming to the rink every day to be around the team and the coaching staff. After I had to stop coaching I would still go on the road some, but being away from the team was difficult for me.

We are working on defining my role with the team going forward. I know that I can do more and that David, Trotzy, and everyone else can rely on me to do whatever it is I can to help. Well, almost anything. I can't go back on the ice ever again, so that is one thing I can't do. Maybe it will help the centers' self-confidence though since they won't all be out there losing faceoffs to me during practice.

After seeing and now being a living and breathing example of what progress the medical profession has made in the treatment of Parkinson's, I am motivated more than ever to do what I can to assist others who have also been dealt this horrible hand in life.

As I have stated before, DBS is not a cure for Parkinson's. I still have it. Unless a breakthrough is made and a cure is found, I will always have Parkinson's.

Making progress in treating and eventually finding a cure for Parkinson's will take many years, but I know that a cure can be found. It will take a lot of research to do so, and that research costs money. A lot of things are known about it, but there are so many other things that we just don't know about yet.

Somewhere, there is a dollar out there that will make the difference and we can find a cure for Parkinson's. I want to find that dollar. With a clear head and a body that is largely responding as it should when I ask it to do something, I am in a good position to dedicate a lot of time and effort to the foundation.

With my last breath and my last step, I promise I will continue to help raise money for Parkinson's patients who live each and every day with this disease. I will also raise money for research and for the caregivers, and do anything I can with the fight against this terrible disease.

In preparing this book, I looked back over my life and am overwhelmed at how blessed I have been. It began with loving and devoted parents who sacrificed a great deal to help me with my quest for a career in hockey. They taught me to live the highest principles of life and to always put those values first and foremost.

Just as I was launching my career, I met and married an incredible young woman who became not only my eternal companion, but also my greatest supporter. She gave me three amazing children. She has had to deal with a lot in their rearing, sometimes alone, given the fact that I was not always there.

The life of a professional athlete is not always easy or glamorous for players and coaches' wives. Tami had to adjust often and needed to be ready at a moment's notice to make major moves and decisions basically on her own. When she was pregnant with Ryan while I was playing in Adirondack, she was having a small problem while shopping and needed my help. This was before cell phones, so she began calling everyone on the team's wife to see if she could find me. She finally found the team captain's wife who informed her that I had been called up to Detroit that very day and was already gone.

When we lived in Vancouver, B.C. she was seven months pregnant with our daughter Kristin. She and the boys were on their way to get haircuts, when over the radio, she heard the news that I had been traded. She did not hear where we were going, only that we were leaving Vancouver.

She had to deal with moving the boys out of school, taking care of transporting the family dog and selling the house while I disappeared from the scene. I told her when I proposed and she accepted that she didn't know what she was in for. For that matter, neither did I.

Hockey has been good for all of us. I have been allowed to make a living by doing what I always loved doing. I have a great family. Ryan and Annie work in a hospital in Atlanta. Brad recently married Amanda and now he has a beautiful stepdaughter named Madalynn. Brad and Amanda have a son on the way as well.

Kristin and Aaron are in New Jersey where Aaron is studying to become a physician's assistant. Tami continues to keep me moving and making sure I keep on the straight and narrow.

Yes, I have been given a serious challenge but I believe that all of us are put upon the earth for a purpose. "Where much is given, much is expected."

I have no idea what my next faceoff will be, but I am determined to continue the game and play by the rules to the best of my ability. I appreciate all of those on my team who keep my back and help me reach the goals that are yet to be made.

Afterword

At the press conference following the conclusion of our 2010-11 season, I made the formal announcement that Brent was no longer going to be a member of our coaching staff in the same capacity as he had since the Nashville Predators came into the National Hockey League. I was very emotional while making the statement and even had to pause a time or two to compose myself in order to get through it.

That day, there were a lot of things that were affecting me. It was about Brent having Parkinson's for sure, but it was also memories of my dad, and the fact that Brent could never fulfill his dream of being an NHL head coach. It was a triple whammy. All those three things were totally in my mind. I had to say the words, but Brent was the one who had to live with it.

My father Norman "Bud" Poile battled Parkinson's for many years. He went through this while Brent and I were working together with the Predators, so Brent knew my dad, saw my dad, and was aware of his fight with Parkinson's from a distance. He saw the devastation the disease caused on my dad. There is some symbolism that Brent now has Parkinson's. From my standpoint, I clearly understand what it is all about, and to this point in time; there is not a cure for it.

I went to Vancouver a lot when my dad was battling Parkinson's. I went along with him to his appointments with his doctors a lot of times. Parkinson's is very frustrating. It is not like you go to the doctor and you lie down on the table and they check out your heart or whatever else may be of concern. The time with the doctors is more about conversations than actual examinations. You are sitting there asking what is wrong with my legs because you can't move them the way that you want to. The doctor says there is nothing wrong with your legs. The Parkinson's causes a disconnect within the body that makes things not work properly.

During his time as a player, I knew a lot about Brent and I always heard good things about him.

The hockey fraternity is pretty small. He had a really good resume of playing and basically went from one day as a player to an assistant coach in the NHL the next day. Brent has the moniker as a student of the game and has always had a really great reputation.

Brent was on everybody's list as an up and coming young coach, so our timing couldn't have been better when we were looking to form our first coaching staff for the Predators. His timing, in his willingness to come here as an assistant coach, was perfect. The interview process was basically a formality for me. You don't have to say too much when you are interviewing Brent. He is such a storyteller, you don't even have to wind him up, he just goes.

The biggest downside on the whole situation in the hockey sense is that Brent never had the opportunity to become a head coach in the NHL. He was clearly on the fast track to become one, and I have no doubt that he would have been a tremendously successful one at that; there are no ands, ifs or buts about it. Prior to Brent's diagnosis, as the years went on, in our meetings at the end of the season I would tell Barry that he better be prepared to lose him. It was just part of our game plan that we were going to lose Brent, but he got thrown a big curve.

Our whole experience in Nashville has been really neat. As I look back, both on and off the ice, and the people I have been fortunate to bring here and hire, they are great hockey people, but more importantly they are great people. There is nobody that is doing as much in the community as the people in our organization. Brent and Barry Trotz are two of the most recognizable people in Nashville right now; A – yes because they are coaches of the Predators, but B – because of everything they do in the community. Maybe B should be A, but either way, they make a difference with not only our hockey team but the community we live in as well.

Parkinson's is terrible, but in the end, the silver lining is that a lot of good has come out of this because Brent and his family have embraced it, going on to do way more than he ever did before. He was a good person and big in the community before, but he has added dimensions to his giving, to his life that I suspect wouldn't have happened if he didn't have this.

Brent is out there even more. Every time you meet him, he leaves an impression because of who he is with the Predators and because he has Parkinson's. He is getting a piece of you because in some way, he is getting you involved. He may not be behind the bench any longer, but he is coaching people up each and every day.

Brent is a great team guy at all times. We all grew up playing hockey and for a lot of us, it is the only job that we have ever had. Barry leans on Brent a lot. As his health dictates, we use him for different things.

After Brent had Deep Brain Stimulation and his condition improved like it did, we had him prescouting the playoffs. That is a pretty big assignment for anybody, but he got that assignment. I am always running things by him… that is if I can catch him.

He has this outgoing personality and wants to be active all the time. Who has more stamina than Brent? He is boundless in his energy whether he is playing golf or doing anything. I don't think he puts much value in being by himself very much. He wants to be with people whether it is with his family or with the hockey guys doing things. That lights him up.

Parkinson's is not the end of the world. There have been big strides medically. When you are really young and are told you have it, it is not great news, but there are no two Parkinson's patients who are alike in terms of their symptoms, how fast it affects them, any number of things. Brent overall has been tracking really well. His attitude has been great and his aggressiveness in treating it has given him more and more opportunities to beat the disease.

It is a disease that I truly believe they can find a cure for. It is there. They have to find something for this. The treatments that Brent has gone through with the DBS, more aggressive and experimental new ideas, you really feel that there is a clear chance that they might be able to find the connection that is missing and finally cure this. All everybody can ask for is hope.

Brent, Tami, and his family have undertaken their Peterson for Parkinson's Foundation, and it has grown in size and donations every year. Let's face it; this is what is going to get everybody to the finish line. This is what is going to find the result.

Printed in Great Britain
by Amazon

20863836R00066